KETO FOR CARB LOVERS COOKBOOK:

1000 DAY QUICK AND EASY KETO CARB LOVERS COOKBOOK THAT WILL MAKE YOUR LIFE EASIER. ENSURE YOUR HEALTHY AND COMFORTABLE COOKING LIFE.

BELINDA TURNER

Table of Contents

Introduction
Chapter 1: Keto Breakfast Recipes
Low-Carb Muffins with Whey
Spinach Rolls
Eggs on Sour Cream
Low-Carb Bacon Muffins
Keto Cheese Tacos
Breakfast Frittata
Keto Waffles
Pumpkin Pancakes
Buttermilk Pancakes
Ricotta Omelet with Swiss Chard
Omelet with Goat Cheese and Herb
Bacon and Zucchini Egg Breakfast
Baked Omelet with Bacon
Egg Keto Cupcakes
Sandwiches With Salad
Keto Avocado with Bacon
Keto Omelet with Mushrooms
Cacao Crunch Cereal
Cheese Shell Breakfast Tacos
Salmon Burrito
Ham Spinach Ballet
Cheesy Thyme Waffles
Keto Low Carb Crepe
Keto Cheese Rolls
Pesto Scramble
Corndogs
Shrimp and Bacon Breakfast
Sausage Patties
Sausage Quiche
Cream Cheese Soufflé
Coconutty Cereal
Cinnamon "Sugar" Cereal"
Keto Mini Doughnuts
Delicious Flax Pancakes
Homemade Bacon and Egg Burgers
Chapter 2: Keto Main Meal Recipes
Lamb Leg with Sun-dried Tomato Pesto
Sirloin with Blue Cheese and Compound Butter
Tuscan Chicken Saute

Garlic Braised Short Ribs
Bacon Wrapped-Beef Tenderloin
Cheeseburger Casserole
Salmon with Mustard Cream
Shrimp and Black Beans Enchalada
Tuna Steaks with Shirataki Noodles
Tilapia with Parmesan Bark
Blackened Fish Tacos with Slaw:
Cheesy Roasted Vegetable Spaghetti
Creamy Chicken & Greens
Curry Chicken Lettuce Wraps
Nacho Chicken Casserole
Pesto & Mozzarella Chicken Casserole
Rotisserie Chicken & Cabbage Shreds
Chicken Quiche
Chicken Parmigiana
Vegetarian Ketogenic Burgers
Tempeh Taco Cups
Mushroom White Pizza
Cheesy Broccoli Nachos with Salsa
One-Skillet Green Pasta
Charred Asparagus with Creamy Sauce
Mozzarella Fish
Cheesy Bacon-Wrapped Chicken with Asparagus Spears
Bacon-Wrapped Chicken with Cheddar Cheese
Delightful Teriyaki Chicken Under Pressure
Turkey and Potatoes with Buffalo Sauce
Happy Burrito Bowl Pork
Sauerkraut Pork
Jalapeno Hash
The Premium Red Pork
Spicy Pork Salad Bowl
Dill and Butter Pork Chops
Cranberry Pork BBQ Dish
Pasta Orecchiette with Broccoli & Tofu
Herbed Portobello Mushrooms
Garlic 'n Sour Cream Zucchini Bake
Paprika 'n Cajun Seasoned Onion Rings
Grilled Parmesan Eggplant
Exquisite Pear and Onion Goose
Turkey Breast with Fennel and Celery
Pancetta and Chicken Risotto
Popcorn Shrimp

Cucumber Ginger Shrimp
Salmon with Pesto
Salmon in Dill Sauce
Flay Beef Empanadas
Basil Halibut Red Pepper Packets
Bistecca Alla Florentina
Zucchini Noodle Beef Lasagna
Chapter 3: Keto Dessert Recipes
Mocha Mousse
Orange Custard Cups
Strawberry Rhubarb Custard
Chocolate Avocado Ice Cream
Key Lime Curd
Coconut Almond Cake
Spicy Almond Fat Bombs
Chocolate Granola Bars
Keto Pumpkin Spice Fat Bombs
Keto Chocolate-Coconut Bites
Blueberry Lemon Cake
Home Made Coconut Ice Cream
Berries with Coconut Cream
Coconut Panna Cotta
Lemon & Lime Sorbet
Keto Vanilla Cherry Panna Cotta
Coconut Flan
Mini Vanilla Custards
Snickerdoodles
Maple Almond Cake in a Jar
Keto Almond Butter Fudge Slices
Almond Flour Shortbread Cookies
Healthy Vanilla-Almond Ice Pops
Low-Carb Raspberry Cheesecake
Keto Lava Cake
Coco Avocado Truffles
Chocolate Chip Cookies
Blueberry Muffins
Peanut Butter Mousse
Cookie Ice Cream
Pumpkin Pecan Ice Cream
Mocha Ice Cream
Conclusion

Table of Contents

INTRODUCTION

CHAPTER 1: KETO BREAKFAST RECIPES

- Low-Carb Muffins with Whey
- Spinach Rolls
- Eggs on Sour Cream
- Low-Carb Bacon Muffins
- Keto Cheese Tacos
- Breakfast Frittata
- Keto Waffles
- Pumpkin Pancakes
- Buttermilk Pancakes
- Ricotta Omelet with Swiss Chard
- Omelet with Goat Cheese and Herb
- Bacon and Zucchini Egg Breakfast
- Baked Omelet with Bacon
- Egg Keto Cupcakes
- Sandwiches With Salad
- Keto Avocado with Bacon
- Keto Omelet with Mushrooms
- Cacao Crunch Cereal
- Cheese Shell Breakfast Tacos
- Salmon Burrito
- Ham Spinach Ballet
- Cheesy Thyme Waffles
- Keto Low Carb Crepe
- Keto Cheese Rolls
- Pesto Scramble
- Corndogs
- Shrimp and Bacon Breakfast
- Sausage Patties
- Sausage Quiche
- Cream Cheese Soufflé
- Coconutty Cereal
- Cinnamon "Sugar" Cereal"
- Keto Mini Doughnuts
- Delicious Flax Pancakes
- Homemade Bacon and Egg Burgers

CHAPTER 2: KETO MAIN MEAL RECIPES

- Lamb Leg with Sun-dried Tomato Pesto
- Sirloin with Blue Cheese and Compound Butter
- Tuscan Chicken Saute
- Garlic Braised Short Ribs
- Bacon Wrapped-Beef Tenderloin
- Cheeseburger Casserole
- Salmon with Mustard Cream
- Shrimp and Black Beans Enchalada
- Tuna Steaks with Shirataki Noodles
- Tilapia with Parmesan Bark
- Blackened Fish Tacos with Slaw:
- Cheesy Roasted Vegetable Spaghetti
- Creamy Chicken & Greens
- Curry Chicken Lettuce Wraps
- Nacho Chicken Casserole
- Pesto & Mozzarella Chicken Casserole
- Rotisserie Chicken & Cabbage Shreds
- Chicken Quiche

Chicken Parmigiana
Vegetarian Ketogenic Burgers
Tempeh Taco Cups
Mushroom White Pizza
Cheesy Broccoli Nachos with Salsa
One-Skillet Green Pasta
Charred Asparagus with Creamy Sauce
Mozzarella Fish
Cheesy Bacon-Wrapped Chicken with Asparagus Spears
Bacon-Wrapped Chicken with Cheddar Cheese
Delightful Teriyaki Chicken Under Pressure
Turkey and Potatoes with Buffalo Sauce
Happy Burrito Bowl Pork
Sauerkraut Pork
Jalapeno Hash
The Premium Red Pork
Spicy Pork Salad Bowl
Dill and Butter Pork Chops
Cranberry Pork BBQ Dish
Pasta Orecchiette with Broccoli & Tofu
Herbed Portobello Mushrooms
Garlic 'n Sour Cream Zucchini Bake
Paprika 'n Cajun Seasoned Onion Rings
Grilled Parmesan Eggplant
Exquisite Pear and Onion Goose
Turkey Breast with Fennel and Celery
Pancetta and Chicken Risotto
Popcorn Shrimp
Cucumber Ginger Shrimp
Salmon with Pesto
Salmon in Dill Sauce
Flay Beef Empanadas
Basil Halibut Red Pepper Packets
Bistecca Alla Florentina
Zucchini Noodle Beef Lasagna
CHAPTER 3: KETO DESSERT RECIPES
Mocha Mousse
Orange Custard Cups
Strawberry Rhubarb Custard
Chocolate Avocado Ice Cream
Key Lime Curd
Coconut Almond Cake
Spicy Almond Fat Bombs
Chocolate Granola Bars
Keto Pumpkin Spice Fat Bombs
Keto Chocolate-Coconut Bites
Blueberry Lemon Cake
Home Made Coconut Ice Cream
Berries with Coconut Cream
Coconut Panna Cotta
Lemon & Lime Sorbet
Keto Vanilla Cherry Panna Cotta
Coconut Flan
Mini Vanilla Custards
Snickerdoodles
Maple Almond Cake in a Jar
Keto Almond Butter Fudge Slices

Almond Flour Shortbread Cookies
Healthy Vanilla-Almond Ice Pops
Low-Carb Raspberry Cheesecake
Keto Lava Cake
Coco Avocado Truffles
Chocolate Chip Cookies
Blueberry Muffins
Peanut Butter Mousse
Cookie Ice Cream
Pumpkin Pecan Ice Cream
Mocha Ice Cream
CONCLUSION

Introduction

The ketogenic diet provides the body with premium fuel in the form of fats that make you fitter and younger with the energy of a twenty-year-old and the best part, and it lasts longer than carb fuel.

By following the ketogenic diet, you can lose all the unwanted weight without ever stepping in a gym without any meal portion control or counting calories. The ketogenic diet has proven to work for people with all types of background and health issues like having blood sugar issues, obesity, post-pregnancy, people having food addictions, those who are suffering from emotional eating, etc. Before going into more detail about the keto diet, let's dive into its history.

The ketogenic diet is nothing new; it has been in existence for over ninety years. Dr. Russell Wilder designed the Keto diet in 1924 as a treatment for his epileptic patients. He found out that fasting that led the body into ketosis proved fruitful to control the epileptic seizures in their patient but fasting wasn't a permanent solution. Hence, they came up with a high-fat and low-carb diet for the patients that worked equally and that too effectively as a cure for epilepsy when no medicine could help. With more research on this diet, the keto diet began being successfully used to treat a variety of other medical conditions, especially obesity. Other benefits apart from epilepsy and losing a few pounds of weights are:

- Alzheimer's disease
- Parkinson's disease
- Multiple Sclerosis
- Healing traumatic brain injuries
- Improve cardiovascular health
- Prevent heart attack and stroke
- Reduce and maintain healthy blood sugar levels
- Fight various kinds of cancer
- Treat Autism
- Decrease acne
- Decrease risk factors for polycystic ovary syndrome and respiratory disease

Our body functions and performs its processes differently at a senior age compared to when it is 20 or 30 years old because, at this age, the metabolism is too slow to burn off any extra calories or fats. Unfortunately, this is a sad reality, but it doesn't mean that a person over 50 cannot implement a ketogenic lifestyle—of course, you can! The ketogenic diet is very varied, and you have to do a few changes in it and adjust to it in a precise way.

Ketogenic diet supports very low or zero-carbs in the diet. And this is not good in the initial days when the body is in the process of transitioning to a Keto Diet. We have always been eating so many carbs that handling this sudden change in the food for our body gets challenging, and you end up suffering from Keto flu. And with more age, your body has a more difficult time adjusting and overcoming the side effects of adapting to the keto diet. The younger generation has a robust support system, but over the age of 50, the side effect hits you harder, and you take more time to recover. You may experience fatigue, headache, nausea, dizziness, lack of motivation, and difficulty focusing. These symptoms are enough to discourage anyone who is finally ready to take charge of their health and body once again, and this stops you from getting the healthy changes you deserve. But don't feel low and worried. Even at this age, the keto diet will work fine for you, and you can still utilize all the incredible benefits of the Ketogenic Diet.

Do you know that eating more fats during a ketogenic diet might prevent you from having a heart stroke? Why? There is a general misconception that fats clog arteries, but that is not the case with the ketogenic diet because you are actually burning fats on the keto diet and losing weight.

Chapter 1: Keto Breakfast Recipes

Low-Carb Muffins with Whey

Preparation Time: 10 minutes
Cooking Time: 30 minutes
Servings: 6
Ingredients:
1 egg
4 tsp. of whey (Chocolate)
4 tbsp. of low-fat milk
1 tsp. of cacao
½ tsp. of vanilla sugar
½ pack of baking powder
Directions:
In one bowl, whisk 1 egg with milk and vanilla sugar. Combine them well.
Gradually, add whey, cacao, and baking powder to the mixture. Mix constantly.
Pour resulting mixture into muffin molds.
Bake at 220°F for 30 minutes. Enjoy!
Nutrition:
Calories: 112
Total Fats: 5g
Net Carbs: 6g
Protein: 1.2g
Fiber: 3.3g

Spinach Rolls

Preparation Time: 10 minutes
Cooking Time: 10 minutes
Servings: 6
Ingredients:
7 oz. of white meat, cut into small cubes
1 cup of spinach
4 eggs
7 oz. of cream cheese
1 tbsp. of sesame seeds
½ tsp. of sodium bicarbonate

4 tbsp. of flour
Directions:
Cook spinach and meat in water. (Separately)
Whisk 3 eggs with 4 tbsp. of flour, sodium, salt, 2 tbsp. of cheese and ½ cup of cooked spinach.
Mix them well and bake at 250°F for 10 minutes.
Meanwhile, dissolve a pinch of salt in water. Add ½ cup of cooked spinach, meat and 1 egg.
Cook the mixture in a cooking pot until meat is done.
Cut baked dough into smaller sizes, fill them with cooked mixture and roll. Enjoy!
Nutrition:
Calories: 123
Total Fats: 4g
Net Carbs: 8g
Protein: 3g
Fiber: 2.4g

Eggs on Sour Cream

Preparation Time: 10 minutes
Cooking Time: 15 minutes
Servings: 6
Ingredients:
6 eggs
1 cup of sour cream
1 tbsp. of parsley
1 tbsp. of butter
Salt, to taste
Directions:
Spread sour cream over casserole dish equally.
Make 6 holes in the sour cream mixture and pour the egg into each one.
Add salt and parsley. Bake for 15 minutes at 250°F.
Nutrition:
Calories: 98
Total Fats: 2g
Net Carbs: 3g
Protein: 4g
Fiber: 5g

Low-Carb Bacon Muffins

Preparation Time: 15 minutes
Cooking Time: 25 minutes
Servings: 6
Ingredients:
2 eggs
4 oz. of sour cream

2 oz. of butter
4 oz. of low-carb flour
4 oz. of cheese
4 oz. of bacon
Salt, to taste
Directions:
Whisk the eggs. Combine them with melted butter, sour cream and flour. Mix well.
Cut bacon thinly. Grind the cheese and then combine these two.
Join 2 mixtures together and fill muffin molds with resulting combination.
Bake for 25 minutes at 220°F. Enjoy!
Nutrition:
Calories: 85
Total Fats: 6g
Net Carbs: 7g
Protein: 2g
Fiber: 6g

Keto Cheese Tacos

Preparation Time: 15 minutes
Cooking Time: 20 minutes
Servings: 6
Ingredients:
3 strips of bacon
1 oz. of cheddar cheese, shredded
½ avocado
2 tbsp. of butter
1 cup of mozzarella cheese, shredded
6 large eggs
Salt and pepper, to taste
Directions:
Start by thoroughly cooking the bacon. Either in an oven for at least 15 to 20 minutes at 375°F or on the stovetop.
Heat a pan in a medium heat and add ⅓ cup of mozzarella.
Cook the cheese until it begins to bubble and turn brown on the side touching the pan. Pay close attention here!
Slip a spatula under the cheese and carefully unstick it from the pan.
Using a pair of tongs, drape the cheese over a wooden spoon, that should be resting over a bowl or pot. Let the cheese to cool and form a taco shell shape.
Repeat Steps 2 to 5 with the remaining mozzarella.
Add the butter and eggs to the pan and cook thoroughly, adding salt and pepper to suit your taste.
Divide the eggs equally between your cheese shells.
Slice the avocado and divide the slices evenly between the tacos.

Chop or crumble your bacon, and divide equally between the tacos.
Sprinkle your cheddar cheese over the tops.
Nutrition:
Calories: 30
Total Fat: 2.5g
Net Carbs: 0.5g
Protein: 1.5g
Fiber: 11.6g

Breakfast Frittata

Preparation Time: 10 minutes
Cooking Time: 30 minutes
Servings: 2
Ingredients:
2 eggs, beaten
2 tbsp. liquid egg whites
2 tbsp. whole ricotta cheese
Pinch sea salt
Pinch ground mustard spice
Pinch black pepper
¼ cup fresh spinach, chopped
2 slices bacon, cooked and crumbled
2 slices tomato
2 tbsp. grated cheese
Directions:
Preheat the oven to 400F. Grease a pie dish.
In a bowl, combine beaten eggs, egg whites, ricotta, sea salt, mustard, and black pepper.
Whisk and beat well.
Add the crumbled bacon and spinach to the mixture and mix.
Pour the egg mixture into the prepared pie dish. Place the tomato slices on top.
Bake for 30 minutes.
Remove from oven and sprinkle with cheese.
Cool, slice, and serve.
Nutrition:
Calories: 116
Fat: 9g
Carb: 1g
Protein: 0g

Keto Waffles

Preparation Time: 5 minutes
Cooking Time: 10 minutes
Servings: 2
Ingredients:

¼ cup almond milk, unsweetened
¼ tsp. apple cider vinegar
1 egg
½ tbsp. olive oil
¼ tsp. vanilla extract
½ cup almond flour
1 tbsp. coconut flour
1 tsp. baking powder
1 tsp. erythritol
Directions:
Preheat the waffle iron and grease it.
In a bowl, mix apple cider vinegar and almond milk.
Add vanilla extract, olive oil, and egg to this mixture. Whisk to combine and set aside.
In another bowl, combine baking powder, coconut flour, almond flour, and erythritol.
Whisk the dry ingredients together.
Combine the dry flour mixture to the wet mixture and whisk to mix.
Pour about ¼ cup batter in the waffle iron.
Cook about three to five minutes until steam stops rising from the waffle iron.
Repeat and serve.
Nutrition:
Calories: 211
Fat: 16g
Carb: 6.5g
Protein: 8g

Pumpkin Pancakes

Preparation Time: 5 minutes
Cooking Time: 12 to 15 minutes
Servings: 2
Ingredients:
1 egg
1 egg white
1 tbsp. cream cheese
1 ½ tbsp. canned pumpkin, unsweetened
½ tbsp. vanilla extract
1/3 cup almond flour
1 tbsp. coconut flour
½ tbsp. Swerve sweetener
½ tsp. pumpkin pie spice
Pinch of salt
½ tsp. baking powder
Pinch of baking soda
¼ tsp. xanthan gum

Water as needed
Directions:
Preheat a griddle to 350F. Add all the wet pancake ingredients except the water to a blender and blend. Now add the dry ingredients.
Continue to blend until smooth.
Add water until pancake batter has the right consistency.
Into the preheated, oiled griddle, pour a small amount of batter.
Cook until browned and the edges almost to the center are dry, about 3 to 4 minutes.
Then flip and heat for 2 to 3 minutes.
Repeat to finish the batter and serve.
Nutrition:
Calories: 230
Fat: 16g
Carb: 9.5g
Protein: 8g

Buttermilk Pancakes

Preparation Time: 5 minutes
Cooking Time: 8 minutes
Servings: 2
Ingredients:
1 ½ tbsp. coconut flour
1 ½ tbsp. almond flour
1 egg
2 tbsp. almond milk + ¼ tsp. apple cider vinegar, mixed in a bowl
¼ tsp. vanilla extract
Pinch of baking powder
½ tsp. erythritol
1 tsp. butter, melted
Pinch of sea salt
Directions:
Mix all the ingredients in a bowl.
Heat a lightly greased skillet over medium-high heat. Make sure the skillet is hot.
Spoon batter onto the skillet and cook until the batter starts to bubble, about 2 minutes.
Then flip and cook until middle is done. Adjust the heat if needed.
Repeat with the remaining batter.
Serve with condiments of choice.
Nutrition:
Calories: 81
Fat: 6g
Carb: 4g
Protein: 3g

Ricotta Omelet with Swiss Chard

Preparation Time: 10 minutes
Cooking Time: 15 minutes
Servings: 2
Ingredients:
6 eggs
2 tbsp. almond milk
½ tsp. kosher salt
½ tsp. ground black pepper
6 tbsp. unsalted butter, divided
2 bunch Swiss chard, cleaned and stemmed
2/3 cup ricotta
Directions:
Add the eggs, and milk. Season with salt and pepper then whisk. Set aside.
In a skillet, melt 4 tbsp. butter. Add the veggie leaves and sauté until just wilted. Remove from pan. Set aside.
Now melt 1 tbsp. butter in the skillet.
Add half of the egg mixture. Spread the mixture. Cook for about 2 minutes.
Add half of the ricotta when the edges are firm, but the center is still a bit runny.
Bend 1/3 of the omelet over the ricotta filling. Transfer to a plate.
Repeat with the remaining butter and egg mixture.
Serve with Swiss chard.
Nutrition:
Calories: 693
Fat: 60g
Carb: 8g
Protein: 2g

Omelet with Goat Cheese and Herb

Preparation Time: 5 minutes
Cooking Time: 12 minutes
Servings: 2
Ingredients:
6 eggs, beaten
2 tbsp. chopped herbs (basil, parsley or cilantro)
Kosher salt and black pepper to taste
2 tbsp. unsalted butter
4 ounces fresh goat cheese
Directions:
Whisk together the eggs, herbs, salt, and pepper.
Melt 1 tbsp. butter in a skillet.
Put half of the egg mixture and cook for 4 to 5 minutes, or until just set.
Crumble half the goat cheese over the eggs and fold in half.
Cook for 1 minute, or until cheese is melted. Transfer to a plate.

Repeat process with the remaining butter, egg mixture, and goat cheese.
Serve.
Nutrition:
Calories: 523
Fat: 43g
Carb: 3g
Protein: 31g

Bacon and Zucchini Egg Breakfast

Preparation Time: 10 minutes
Cooking Time: 10 minutes
Servings: 2
Ingredients:
2 cups zucchini noodles
2 slices of raw bacon
¼ cup grated Asiago cheese
2 eggs
Salt and pepper to taste
Directions :
Cut the bacon slices into ¼ inch thick strips.
Cook the bacon in a pan for 3 minutes.
Add the zucchini and mix well.
Season with salt and pepper.
Flatten slightly with a spatula and make 2 depressions for the eggs.
Sprinkle with the cheese.
Break one egg into each dent.
Cook 3 minutes more, then cover and cook for 2 to 4 minutes, or until the eggs are cooked.
Serve.
Nutrition:
Calories: 242
Fat: 19g
Carb: 4g
Protein: 14g

Baked Omelet with Bacon

Preparation Time: 5 minutes
Cooking Time: 30 minutes
Servings: 1
Ingredients:
4 eggs
140 g diced bacon
85 g butter
60 g fresh spinach
1 tbsp. l finely chopped fresh onions (to taste)

salt and pepper
Directions:
Preheat the oven to 400 ° F. Oil one small baking dish (per serving).
Fry the bacon and spinach in the remaining oil.
In another bowl, whisk the eggs until it's foamy. Mix the bacon and spinach, gradually adding the fat remaining after frying the products.
Then add finely chopped onions. Flavor the dish with salt and pepper.
Put the mixture into a baking sheet then bake for at least 20 minutes or until golden brown.
Recover the dish and let it cool for a few minutes. After that, you can serve.
Nutrition:
Carbohydrates: 12 g
Fats: 72 g
Proteins: 21 g
Calories: 737

Egg Keto Cupcakes

Preparation Time: 10 minutes
Cooking Time: 25 minutes
Servings: 6
Ingredients:
2 pcs green onions finely chopped green onions
150 g Sausages of sliced sausages or bacon
12 pcs Egg
2 tbsp. l Pesto
Salt and pepper
175 g grated cheese
Directions:
Preheat the oven to 350 ° F.
Lubricate the muffin pan with butter.
Fill onions and sausages at the bottom of the molds.
Beat the eggs with pesto, salt, and pepper. Add cheese and mix thoroughly.
Fill the cupcake pan with the resulting mixture.
Bake in the oven for 15-20 minutes depending on the size of the mold.
Nutrition:
Carbohydrates: 2 g
Fats: 26 g
Proteins: 23 g
Kcal: 336

Sandwiches With Salad

Preparation Time: 5 minutes
Cooking Time: 0 minutes
Servings: 1
Ingredients:

50 g Roman salad
15 g Butter
30 g Cheese of Eden cheese or other cheese (to your taste)
0.5 pcs Avocado
1 pc cherry tomato
Directions:
Rinse the lettuce leaves thoroughly and use them as a base for the filling.
Oil the leaves, chop the cheese, avocado, and tomato and place on the leaves.
Nutrition:
Fats: 34 g
Proteins: 10 g
Carbohydrates: 3 g
Calories: 374

Keto Avocado with Bacon

Preparation Time: 5 minutes
Cooking Time: 20 minutes
Servings: 1
Ingredients:
4 hard-boiled egg
1 pc avocado
2 tbsp. olive oil
100 g bacon
salt and pepper
Directions:
Preheat oven to 350 ° F.
In a pan that filled of water, put the egg. Set to a boil and let it brew for 8-10 minutes. Place the eggs in ice water immediately after preparation to make them easier to clean.
Cut the eggs in half and dig up the yolks. Place them in a small bowl.
Add avocado, butter, and mashed potatoes until salt and pepper are mixed to taste.
Set the bacon on a baking sheet then bake until crispy. It takes about 5-7 minutes.
Using a spoon, carefully add the mixture back to the cooked egg whites and set the sails with bacon! Enjoy it!
Nutrition:
Pure carbohydrates: 1 g
Fats: 13 g
Proteins: 5 g
Calories: 144

Keto Omelet with Mushrooms

Preparation Time: 5 minutes
Cooking Time: 10 minutes
Servings: 1
Ingredients:

3 eggs
30 g butter for frying
30 g (60 ml) grated cheese
$^1/_5$ onion
3 pcs. mushrooms
salt and pepper
Directions:
Break the eggs then put the contents into a small bowl.
Add salt and pepper to taste.
Beat the eggs with a fork until a uniform foam is formed.
In a pan, heat a piece of butter, and as soon as the butter has melted, pour the egg mixture into the pan.
When the mixture begins to harden and fry, and the eggs on top will still be liquid, sprinkle them with cheese, mushrooms, and onions (to taste).
Take a spatula and gently pry the edges of the omelet on one side, and then fold the omelet in half. As soon as the dish begins to take a golden brownish tint, remove the pan from the stove then place the omelet on a plate.
Nutrition:
Carbohydrates: 5 g
Fats: 44 g
Proteins: 26 g
Kcal: 649

Cacao Crunch Cereal

Preparation Time: 5 minutes
Cooking Time: 0 minutes
Servings: 2
Ingredients:
½ cup slivered almonds
2 tablespoons coconut, shredded or flakes
2 tablespoons chia seeds
2 tablespoons cacao nibs
2 tablespoons sunflower seeds
Unsweetened nondairy milk of choice (I use macadamia milk), for serving
Directions:
In a small bowl, mix the almonds, coconut, chia seeds, cacao nibs, and sunflower seeds.
Divide between two bowls.
Pour in the nondairy milk and serve.
Nutrition:
Calories: 325
Total Fat: 27
Protein: 10g
Total Carbs: 17g

Fiber: 12g
Net Carbs: 5g

Cheese Shell Breakfast Tacos

Preparation Time: 10 minutes
Cooking Time: 15 minutes
Servings: 2
Ingredients:
1⅓ cups shredded Mexican blend cheese
1 tablespoon butter or ghee
4 large eggs
2 tablespoons heavy whipping cream
Salt
Freshly ground black pepper
Dash hot sauce
1 avocado, pitted, peeled, and sliced or cubed
1 tablespoon chopped cilantro
Directions:
Preheat the oven to 350°F. Line a baking sheet using a silicone baking mat or parchment paper.
Add ⅓-cup mounds of shredded cheese to the pan, leaving plenty of space between them. Bake until the each sides are brown and the middle of each has fully melted, about 7 minutes.
Set the pan on the cooking rack. You will need to move quickly to bend the shells while they are still pliable. You can get creative with what you want to bend them over. I like to create a "rack" over my sink with a wider cooling rack to drape them over or sometimes over the sides of a larger storage container. As they cool, they will harden.
In a skillet, heat the butter at medium heat.
Whisk in the eggs and heavy cream, and season with salt, pepper, and a dash of hot sauce. Scramble the eggs for 3 minutes, or to desired doneness.
Fill the cheese shells with the scrambled eggs, and top with the avocado and cilantro.
Nutrition:
Calories: 661
Total Fat: 57g
Protein: 33g
Total Carbs: 8g
Fiber: 5g
Net Carbs: 3g

Salmon Burrito

Preparation Time: 6 minutes
Cooking Time: 4 minutes
Servings: 2
Ingredients:

For base and flavor:
Chopped chives, a pinch
Dried cumin and coriander, a pinch
Chopped rosemary, a pinch
Salt and pepper to taste
2 Eggs, (to form a burrito roll)
Oil for frying the eggs
For filling:
½ Avocado, (chunks)
½ cup Salmon, (cooked/boiled)
¼ cup Spinach, (cooked/boiled)
Directions:
Pick a pan and warm the oil over medium heat.
Mix the egg in a bowl with salt and pepper.
Combine the chives, rosemary, cumin, and coriander in the beaten egg.
Fry the egg and spread each on a separate plate after cooking.
Place the filling over the eggs spread on the plates; equally divide the avocado, spinach, salmon.
Roll the eggs with filling to form in a burrito and serve.
Nutrition:
Calories: 331
Fat: 30 g
Fiber: 3 g
Carbs: 10 g
Net Carbs: 7 g
Protein: 11 g

Ham Spinach Ballet

Preparation Time: 10 minutes
Cooking Time: 30 minutes
Servings: 2
Ingredients:
4 teaspoons cream
¾ pound fresh baby spinach
7-ounce ham, sliced
Salt and black pepper, to taste
1 tablespoon unsalted butter, melted
Directions:
Set the oven to 360°F and grease 2 ramekins with butter.
Put butter and spinach in a skillet and cook for about 3 minutes.
Add cooked spinach in the ramekins and top with ham slices, cream, salt and black pepper.
Bake for about 25 minutes and dish out to serve hot.

For meal prepping, you can refrigerate this ham spinach ballet for about 3 days wrapped in a foil.

Nutrition

Calories:188

Fat: 12.5g

Carbs: 4.9g

Protein: 14.6g

Sugar: 0.3g

Cheesy Thyme Waffles

Preparation Time: 5 minutes

Cooking Time: 10 minutes

Servings: 2

Ingredients:

½ cup mozzarella cheese, finely shredded

¼ cup Parmesan cheese

¼ large head cauliflower

½ cup collard greens

1 large egg

1 stalk green onion

½ tablespoon olive oil

½ teaspoon garlic powder

¼ teaspoon salt

½ tablespoon sesame seed

1 teaspoon fresh thyme, chopped

¼ teaspoon ground black pepper

Directions:

Put cauliflower, collard greens, spring onion and thyme in a food processor and pulse until smooth.

Put mixture in a bowl and mix in rest of the ingredients.

Heat a waffle iron and transfer the mixture evenly over the griddle.

Cook until a waffle is formed and dish out in a serving platter.

Nutrition:

Calories: 144

Carbs: 8.5g

Fats: 9.4g

Proteins: 9.3g

Sodium: 435mg

Sugar: 3g

Keto Low Carb Crepe

Preparation Time: 5 minutes

Cooking Time: 8 minutes

Servings: 2

Ingredients:
2 eggs
1 egg white
1 tbsp. unsalted butter
1 1/3 tbsp. cream cheese
2/3 tbsp. psyllium husk
Directions:
Prepare the batter and for this, put all the ingredients in a bowl, except for butter, and then whisk by using a stick blender until smooth and very liquid.
Bring out a skillet pan, put it over medium heat, add ½ tbsp. butter and when it melts, pour in half of the batter, spread evenly, and cook until the top has firmed.
Carefully flip the crepe, then continue cooking for 2 minutes until cooked and then move it to a plate.
Put the remaining butter then when it melts, cook another crepe in the same manner and then serve.
Nutrition:
Calories: 118
Fats: 7 g
Protein: 1g
Carbohydrates: 1 g

Keto Cheese Rolls

Preparation Time: 5 minutes
Cooking Time: 0 minutes
Servings: 2
Ingredients:
1-oz butter, unsalted
2 oz. mozzarella cheese, sliced, full-fat
Directions:
Cut cheese into slices and then cut butter into thin slices.
Top each cheese slice with a slice of butter, roll it and then serve.
Nutrition:
Calories: 166
Fats: 7g
Protein: 2 g
Carbohydrates: 0 g

Pesto Scramble

Preparation Time: 5 minutes
Cooking Time: 5 minutes
Servings: 2
Ingredients:
1 tbsp. basil pesto
1 tbsp. unsalted butter

1/8 tsp ground black pepper
1/8 tsp salt
2 eggs
2 tbsp. grated cheddar cheese
Directions:
Crack eggs in a bowl, add cheese, black pepper, salt, and pesto and whisk until combined. Bring out a skillet pan, put it over medium heat, add the butter and when it melts, add in the egg mixture and cook for 3 to 5 min until eggs have scrambled to the desired level.
Nutrition:
Calories: 160
Fats: 7g
Protein: 2 g
Carbohydrates: 0 g

Corndogs

Preparation Time: 15 minutes
Cooking Time: 12 minutes
Servings: 4
Ingredients:
1 tsp baking powder
¼ tsp cayenne pepper
1 cup almond meal
½ tsp turmeric
1 tsp Italian seasoning
Salt and ground black pepper to taste
2 tbsp heavy cream
2 eggs
4 sausages
1½ cups olive oil
Directions:
In a medium bowl, mix together baking powder, cayenne pepper, almond meal, turmeric, Italian seasoning, salt and pepper. Set aside.
In another bowl, whisk together heavy cream and eggs.
Pour egg mixture into almond meal mixture and stir to combine.
Toss sausages in bowl until they are covered in mixture.
Pour oil in pan and preheat over medium-high heat.
Transfer sausages to pan and cook for 2 minutes per side.
Place cooked sausages on plate, drain grease and serve.
Nutrition:
Calories 340
Carbs 5.2g
Fat 32g
Protein 16.7g

Shrimp and Bacon Breakfast

Preparation Time: 15 minutes
Cooking Time: 17 minutes
Servings: 4
Ingredients:
1 cup mushrooms
4 bacon slices
4 oz. smoked salmon, chopped
4 oz. shrimp, deveined
Salt and ground black pepper to taste
½ cup coconut cream
Directions:
Preheat pan over medium heat.
Meanwhile, chop bacon. Put bacon to pan and cook for 5 minutes.
Slice mushrooms and add to pan, cook for another 5 minutes, stirring occasionally.
Add salmon and stir. Cook for 3 minutes more.
Add shrimp and stir. Cook for 2 minutes more.
Sprinkle with salt and pepper, stir.
Add coconut cream, stir and cook for another 1 minute.
Serve warm.
Nutrition:
Calories 335
Carbs 4.2g
Fat 24g
Protein 17.5g

Sausage Patties

Preparation Time: 15 minutes
Cooking Time: 12 minutes
Servings: 2
Ingredients:
1 lb. minced pork
Salt and ground black pepper to taste
½ tsp sage, dried
¼ tsp thyme, dried
¼ tsp ground ginger
3 tbsp. cold water
1 tbsp. coconut oil
Directions:
In small bowl, combine salt, sage, pepper, thyme, ginger and water.
In medium bowl, combine spice mix with pork.
Make patties and set aside.
Add coconut oil to pan and preheat it on medium high heat.

Transfer patties to pan and cook for 5 minutes, then flip, and cook them for 3 minutes more.
Serve.
Nutrition:
Calories 318
Carbs 11g
Fat 12.8g
Protein 11.8g

Sausage Quiche

Preparation Time: 15 minutes
Cooking Time: 45 minutes
Servings: 6
Ingredients:
12 oz. pork sausage
5 eggplants
10 mixed cherry tomatoes, halved
6 eggs, beaten
2 tsp whipping cream
2 tbsp. Parmesan cheese, grated
2 tbsp. fresh parsley, chopped
Salt and ground black pepper to taste
Directions:
Chop sausage and place on the bottom of a baking dish.
Slice eggplants and lay on top.
Lay cherry tomatoes on eggplant.
In a medium bowl, put and combine eggs, cream, Parmesan cheese, parsley, salt and pepper.
Pour mixture over tomatoes.
Preheat oven to 375 F.
Set the baking dish in oven and cook for 40 minutes.
Top with parsley and serve.
Nutrition:
Calories 338
Carbs 2.9g
Fat 27.5g
Protein 17.1g

Cream Cheese Soufflé

Preparation Time: 15 minutes
Cooking Time: 20 minutes
Servings: 4
Ingredients:
1/3 cup spinach, chopped roughly

1 tsp coconut oil
¼ cup white onion, peeled and diced
1 egg, beaten
½ cup cream cheese
¼ cup coconut flour
1 tsp salt
1 tsp paprika
Directions:
Place spinach in blender or food processor and blend until texture smooth.
Preheat pan with coconut oil on medium heat.
Add onion and sauté for about 5 minutes, stirring constantly, until onion turn golden brown.
In medium bowl, combine egg, cream cheese and coconut flour.
Season mixture with salt and paprika, stir well.
Add cooked onion to mixture and stir.
Pour soufflé in baking dish.
Place dish in oven at 365 F and bake for 10 minutes
Remove baking dish from oven and whisk it carefully. Serve.
Nutrition:
Calories 196
Carbs 5.3g
Fat 16.9g
Protein 5.6g

Coconutty Cereal

Preparation Time: 5 minutes
Cooking Time: 5 minutes
Servings: 2
Ingredients:
1 cup coconut, shredded or flakes
1 teaspoon erythritol
Unsweetened nondairy milk of choice (I use macadamia milk), for serving
Directions:
.Preheat the oven to 350°F.
On a baking sheet, arrange the coconut flakes in a single layer.
Bake for about 5 minutes, until nice and golden.
Allow the coconut flakes cool for around 5 to 10 minutes, then toss them with the erythritol in a plastic ziptop bag and shake.
Divide between two bowls and pour in the nondairy milk. Serve.
Nutrition:
Calories: 247
Total Fat: 24g
Protein: 3g

Total Carbs: 7g
Fiber: 6g
Net Carbs: 1g

Cinnamon “Sugar” Cereal”

Preparation Time: 5 minutes
Cooking Time: 10 minutes
Servings: 2
Ingredients:
1 cup coconut, shredded or flakes
2 tablespoons butter or ghee
1 tablespoon ground cinnamon
1 teaspoon erythritol
2 tablespoons cacao nibs
Unsweetened nondairy milk of choice (I use macadamia milk), for serving
Directions:
Preheat the oven to 325°F.
Bring the coconut flakes in a small bowl.
In a saucepan, add the butter, cinnamon, and erythritol over medium heat, melt, and mix well.
Pour the mixture in the coconut flakes, stir to mix, then put the coated coconut flakes on the baking dish.
Bake for at least 5 to 7 minutes, or until nice and golden. Stir the coconut flakes a couple of times to toast all sides and make sure they don’t burn.
Allow the coconut flakes cool for 5 to 10 minutes.
Divide between two bowls, add the cacao nibs, and pour in the nondairy milk to serve.
Nutrition:
Calories: 405
Total Fat: 40g
Protein: 4g
Total Carbs: 12g
Fiber: 10g
Net Carbs: 2g

Keto Mini Doughnuts

Preparation Time: 15 minutes
Cooking Time: 10 minutes
Servings: 22
Ingredients:
4 tbsp. almond flour
1 tbsp. coconut flour
1 tsp. vanilla extract
1 tsp. baking powder
4 tbsp. erythritol

3 oz. cream cheese
3 large eggs
10 drops liquid stevia
Directions:
Combine with an immersion blender or a food processor.
Make sure that all your ingredients are well blended and smooth.
Heat your doughnut maker and spray with your grease of choice. Coconut oil always gives your cooking a delicious finish!
Pour your mixture into the doughnut maker. Leave some room (say 10%) to give your doughnuts space to rise.
Let the mixture cook for 3 minutes, and then flip and cook for an additional 2 minutes.
Remove the baked doughnuts and repeat Steps 3 to 5 for the rest of your batter.
Nutrition:
Calories: 30
Total Fat: 2.5g
Net Carbs: 0.5g
Protein: 1.5g
Fiber: 11.6g

Delicious Flax Pancakes

Preparation Time: 5 minutes
Cooking Time: 20 minutes
Servings: 3
Ingredients:
150 g of fat sour cream
4 eggs
½ tsp. of salt
1 tsp. of baking powder
50 g of room temperature butter
6 tsp. with a hill of ground flax seeds
sweetener to taste
20 g of any fat for frying
Directions:
Using a mixer, beat the butter, add the eggs, sour cream, baking powder, salt, and sweetener and beat until smooth all together
Add one spoonful of flax and continue to whisk.
The dough should turn out as it is for pancakes, that is, as a thick sour cream.
Heat the pan, put the oil in and fry as usual. But layout the circles thickly and with a diameter of about 4 cm, because they sprawl out and become larger.
Fry over low heat, otherwise they will burn.
Nutrition:
Carbohydrates: 1.42 g
Fats: 7.20 g

Proteins: 2.08 g
Calories: 75.69

Homemade Bacon and Egg Burgers

Preparation Time: 10 minutes
Cooking Time: 30 minutes
Servings: 3
Ingredients:
6 eggs
3 tbsp. of nutmeg, I used peanut
50 g of butter, melted
salt, black pepper to taste
Ingredients for the filling
9 strips of bacon
3 eggs
Directions:
Mix the ingredients for the pancakes and fry as usual. To make them perfectly round, it is better to use silicone molds for pancakes or scrambled eggs.
Fry three eggs. It is advisable to use forms too.
Fry the bacon.
Combine all the ingredients in the form of a burger, in addition, use everything you want: herbs, cucumbers, cheese or salsa sauce.
Nutrition:
Carbohydrates: 3.2 g
Fats: 35.8 g
Proteins: 26.78 g
Calories: 447.62

Chapter 2: Keto Main Meal Recipes

Lamb Leg with Sun-dried Tomato Pesto

Preparation Time: 15 minutes
Cooking Time: 70 minutes
Servings: 8
Ingredients:
For the Pesto:
1 cup sun-dried tomatoes packed in oil
¼ cup pine nuts
2 tablespoons extra-virgin olive oil
2 tablespoons chopped fresh basil
2 teaspoons minced garlic
For the Lamb Leg:
1 (2-pound) lamb leg
Sea salt
Freshly ground black pepper

2 tablespoons olive oil
Directions:
To make the Pesto:
Place the sun-dried tomatoes, pine nuts, olive oil, basil, and garlic in a blender or food processor; process until smooth.
Set aside until needed.
To make the Lamb Leg
Preheat the oven to 400°F.
Season the lamb leg all over with salt and pepper.
Bring a large ovenproof skillet over medium-high heat and add the olive oil.
Sear the lamb on all sides until nicely browned, about 6 minutes in total.
Spread the sun-dried tomato pesto all over the lamb and place the lamb on a baking sheet.
Roast
Let the lamb rest for 10 minutes before slicing and serving.
Nutrition:
Calories: 352
Fat: 29g
Protein: 17g
Carbs: 5g
Fiber: 2g
Net Carbs: 3g

Sirloin with Blue Cheese and Compound Butter

Preparation Time: 10 minutes
Cooking Time: 12 minutes
Servings: 4
Ingredients:
6 tablespoons butter, at room temperature
4 oz. blue cheese
4 (5-ounce) beef sirloin steaks
1 tablespoon olive oil
Sea salt
Freshly ground black pepper
Directions:
Place the butter in a blender and pulse until the butter is whipped, about 2 minutes.
Add the cheese and pulse until just incorporated.
Spoon the butter mixture onto a sheet of plastic wrap and roll it into a log about 1½ inches in diameter by twisting both ends of the plastic wrap in opposite directions.
Refrigerate the butter until completely set, about 1 hour.
Slice the butter into ½-inch disks and set them on a plate in the refrigerator until you are ready to serve the steaks. Keep leftover butter in the fridge for up to 1 week.
Preheat a barbecue to medium-high heat.
Let the steaks come to room temperature.

Rub the steaks all over with the olive oil and season them with salt and pepper.
Grill the steaks until they reach your desired doneness, about 6 minutes per side for medium.
If you don't have a barbecue, broil the steaks in a preheated oven for 7 minutes per side for medium.
Let the steaks rest for 10 minutes. Serve each topped with a disk of the compound butter.
Nutrition:
Calories: 544
Fat: 44g
Protein: 35g
Carbs: 0g
Fiber: 0g
Net Carbs: 0g

Tuscan Chicken Saute

Preparation Time: 10 minutes
Cooking Time: 35 minutes
Servings: 4
Ingredients:
1 pound boneless chicken breasts, each cut into three pieces
Sea salt, for seasoning
Freshly ground black pepper, for seasoning
3 tablespoons olive oil
1 tablespoon minced garlic
¾ cup chicken stock
1 teaspoon dried oregano
½ teaspoon dried basil
½ cup heavy (whipping) cream
½ cup shredded Asiago cheese
1 cup fresh spinach
¼ cup sliced Kalamata olives
Directions:
Prepare the chicken. Pat, the chicken, breasts dry and lightly season them with salt and pepper.
Sauté the chicken. In a large skillet over medium-high heat, warm the olive oil. Add the chicken and sauté until it is golden brown and just cooked through, about 15 minutes in total. Transfer the chicken to a plate and set it aside.
Make the sauce. Put the garlic to the skillet, then sauté until it's softened about 2 minutes. Stir in the chicken stock, oregano, and basil, scraping up any browned bits in the skillet. Bring to a boil, then reduce the heat to low and simmer until the sauce is reduced by about one-quarter, about 10 minutes.
Finish the dish. Stir in the cream, Asiago, and simmer, stirring the sauce frequently, until it has thickened about 5 minutes. Put back the chicken to the skillet along with any

accumulated juices. Stir in the spinach and olives and simmer until the spinach is wilted about 2 minutes.
Serve. Divide the chicken and sauce between four plates and serve it immediately.
Nutrition:
Calories: 483
Total fat: 38g
Total carbs: 5g
Fiber: 1g;
Net carbs: 3g
Sodium: 332mg
Protein: 31g

Garlic Braised Short Ribs

Preparation Time: 10 minutes
Cooking Time: 2 hours and 20 minutes
Servings: 10
Ingredients:
4 (4-ounce) beef short ribs
Sea salt
Freshly ground black pepper
1 tablespoon olive oil
2 teaspoons minced garlic
½ cup dry red wine
3 cups Rich Beef Stock
Directions:
Preheat the oven to 325°F.
Season the beef ribs on each side with salt and pepper.
Set a deep ovenproof skillet at medium-high heat and add the olive oil.
Sear the ribs per side until browned, about 6 minutes in total. Transfer the ribs to a plate.
Put the garlic to the skillet and sauté until translucent, about 3 minutes.
Mix in the red wine to deglaze the pan. Ensure to scrape all the browned bits from the meat from the bottom of the pan. Simmer the wine until it is slightly reduced for at least 2 minutes.
Pour the beef stock, ribs, and any accumulated juices on the plate back to the skillet and bring the liquid to a boil.
Cover the skillet and bring it in the oven to braise the ribs until the meat is fall-off-the-bone tender, about 2 hours.
Serve the ribs with a spoonful of the cooking liquid drizzled over each serving.
Nutrition:
Calories: 481
Fat: 38g
Protein: 29g
Carbs: 5g

Fiber: 3g
Net Carbs: 2g

Bacon Wrapped-Beef Tenderloin

Preparation Time: 10 minutes
Cooking Time: 15 minutes
Servings: 4
Ingredients:
4 (4-ounce) beef tenderloin steaks
Sea salt
Freshly ground black pepper
8 bacon slices
1 tablespoon extra-virgin olive oil
Directions:
Preheat the oven to 450°F.
Season the steaks with salt and pepper.
Wrap each steak snugly around the edges with 2 slices of bacon and secure the bacon with toothpicks.
Bring a large skillet at medium-high heat and add the olive oil.
Pan sear the steaks for 4 minutes per side and transfer them to a baking sheet.
Roast the steaks until they reach your desired doneness, about 6 minutes for medium.
Remove the steaks from the oven and let them rest for 10 minutes.
Remove the toothpicks and serve.
Nutrition:
Calories: 565
Fat: 49g
Protein: 28g
Carbs: 0g
Fiber: 0g
Net Carbs: 0g

Cheeseburger Casserole

Preparation Time: 10 minutes
Cooking Time: 40 minutes
Servings: 6
Ingredients:
1 pound 75% lean ground beef
½ cup chopped sweet onion
2 teaspoons minced garlic
1½ cups shredded aged Cheddar, divided
½ cup heavy (whipping) cream
1 large tomato, chopped
1 teaspoon minced fresh basil
¼ teaspoon sea salt

⅛ teaspoon freshly ground black pepper
Directions:
Preheat the oven to 350°F.
Set a large skillet at medium-high heat and add the ground beef.
Brown the beef until cooked through, about 6 minutes, and spoon off any excess fat.
Stir in the onion and garlic and cook until the vegetables are tender about 4 minutes.
Transfer the beef and vegetables to an 8-by-8-inch casserole dish.
In a medium bowl, place 1 cup of shredded cheese and the heavy cream, tomato, basil, salt, and pepper then mix until well combined.
Pour the cream mixture over the beef mixture and top the casserole with the remaining ½ cup of shredded cheese.
Bake until the casserole is bubbly and the cheese is melted and lightly browned, about 30 minutes.
Serve.
Nutrition:
Calories: 410
Fat: 33g
Protein: 20g
Carbs: 3g
Fiber: 0g
Net Carbs: 3g

Salmon with Mustard Cream

Preparation Time: 10 minutes
Cooking Time: 12 minutes
Servings: 2
Ingredients:
2 salmon fillets
¼ cup keto mayo
1 tbsp. Dijon mustard
2 tbsp. fresh cilantro, minced
2 tbsp. ghee butter
½ tsp garlic powder
Salt and pepper to taste
Directions:
Preheat the oven to 450F. Grease a baking dish with the ghee butter
Season the salmon with salt and pepper and put in the baking dish
In a mixing bowl, put and combine the Dijon mustard, mayo, parsley, and garlic powder. Stir well
Top the salmon fillets with the mustard sauce
Bake for 10 minutes
Nutrition:
Carbs: 2 g

Fat: 41,5 g
Protein: 32,9 g
Calories: 505

Shrimp and Black Beans Enchalada

Preparation Time: 5 minutes
Cooking Time: 15 minutes
Servings: 4
Ingredients:
2 cans (10 g) of red or green enchilada sauce
1 lb. shrimp
2 cans (15 oz.) black beans
2 cups grated Mexican cheese mixture
12 to 13 small flour tortillas
Directions:
Preheat the oven to 400° F. Put ¼ cup sauce (enchiladas) in a saucepan. Increase the heat and add the shrimp. Cook until the shrimp are clean and no longer transparent for about 5 minutes. Remove from the heated container.
Place the enchiladas in a 9 x 13-inch baking dish. Organize a pea breakfast, 3 or 4 shrimp, and a slice of cheese on an omelet. Fold the tortilla edges into the oven dish on the filling and with the seam facing down.
Repeat with the remaining tortillas. Pour out the rest of the enchilada sauce after preparing all the enchiladas.
Bake until all the cheese has melted for 15 minutes.
Nutrition:
Calories: 196
Fat: 12g
Net Carbs: 4g
Protein: 17g

Tuna Steaks with Shirataki Noodles

Preparation Time: 10 minutes
Cooking Time: 20 minutes
Servings: 4
Ingredients:
1 pack (7 oz.) miracle noodle angel hair
3 cups water
1 red bell pepper, seeded and halved
4 tuna steaks
Salt and black pepper to taste
Olive oil for brushing
2 tablespoons pickled ginger
2 tablespoons chopped cilantro
Directions:

Cook the shirataki rice based on the package instructions: In a colander, rinse the shirataki noodles with running cold water.
Place a pot of salted water to a boil; blanch the noodles for 2 minutes.
Drain and moved to a dry skillet over medium heat.
Dry roast for a few minutes until opaque.
Grease a grill's grate using a cooking spray and preheat on medium heat. Spice the red bell pepper and tuna with salt and black pepper, brush with olive oil, and grill covered.
Cook both for at least 3 minutes on each side. Moved to a plate to cool. Dice bell pepper with a knife.
Arrange the noodles, tuna, and bell pepper into the serving plate.
Top with pickled ginger and garnish with cilantro.
Serve with roasted sesame sauce.
Nutrition:
Calories: 310
Fat: 18.2g
Net Carbs: 2g
Protein: 22g

Tilapia with Parmesan Bark

Preparation Time: 4 minutes
Cooking Time: 12 minutes
Servings: 4
Ingredients:
¾ cup freshly grated Parmesan cheese
2 teaspoons pepper
1 tablespoon chopped parsley
4 tilapia fillets (4 us)
Lemon cut into pieces
Directions:
Set the oven to 400° F. Mix cheese in a shallow dish with pepper and parsley and season with salt and pepper.
Mix the fish in the cheese with olive oil and flirt. Place on a baking sheet with foil and bake for 10 to 12 minutes until the fish in the thickest part is opaque.
Serve the lemon slices with the fish.
Nutrition:
Calories: 210
Fat: 9.3g
Net Carbs: 1.3g
Protein: 28.9g

Blackened Fish Tacos with Slaw:

Preparation Time: 14 minutes
Cooking Time: 6 minutes
Servings: 4

Ingredients:
1 tablespoon olive oil
1 teaspoon chili powder
2 tilapia fillets
1 teaspoon paprika
4 low carb tortillas
Slaw:
½ cup red cabbage, shredded
1 tablespoon lemon juice
1 teaspoon apple cider vinegar
1 tablespoon olive oil
Salt and black pepper to taste
Directions:
Season the tilapia with chili powder and paprika. Heat the vegetable oil during a skillet over medium heat.
Add tilapia and cook until blackened, about 3 minutes per side. Cut into strips. Divide the tilapia between the tortillas. Blend all the slaw ingredients in a bowl and top the fish to serve.
Nutrition:
Calories: 268
Fat: 20g
Net Carbs: 3.5g
Protein: 13.8g

Cheesy Roasted Vegetable Spaghetti

Preparation Time: 10 minutes
Cooking Time: 35 minutes
Servings: 4
Ingredients:
2 (8 oz.) packs shirataki spaghetti
1 cup chopped mixed bell peppers
½ cup grated Parmesan cheese for topping
1 lb. asparagus, chopped
1 cup broccoli florets
1 cup green beans, chopped
3 tbsp. olive oil
1 small onion, chopped
2 garlic cloves, minced
1 cup diced tomatoes
½ cup chopped basil
Directions:
Boil 2 cups water in a pot. Strain the shirataki pasta and rinse well under hot running water. Allow draining and pour the shirataki pasta into the boiling water. Cook for 3

minutes and strain again. Place a dry skillet and stir-fry the shirataki pasta until visibly dry, 1-2 minutes; set aside. Preheat oven to 425°F. In a bowl, add asparagus, broccoli, bell peppers, and green beans and toss with half of the olive oil. Bring the vegetables on a baking sheet and roast for 20 minutes. Heat the remaining olive oil in a skillet and sauté onion and garlic for 3 minutes. Stir in tomatoes and cook for 8 minutes. Mix in shirataki and vegetables. Top with Parmesan cheese and serve.

Nutrition:

Calories 272

Net Carbs 7g

Fats 12g

Protein 12g

Creamy Chicken & Greens

Preparation Time: 10 minutes

Cooking Time: 20 minutes

Servings: 4

Ingredients:

1 lb. Chicken thighs – skins on

1 cup. Chicken stock

1 cup. Cream

2 tbsp. Coconut oil

1 tsp. Italian herbs

2 cups Dark leafy greens

Pepper & Salt (your preference)

2 tbsp. Coconut flour

2 tbsp. Melted butter

Directions:

On the stovetop, add oil in a skillet using the med-high temperature setting.

Remove the bones from the chicken and dust using salt and pepper. Fry the chicken until done.

Make the sauce by adding the butter to a saucepan. Whisk in the flour to form a thick paste. Slowly, whisk in the cream. Once it boils, mix in the herbs.

Transfer the chicken to the counter and add the stock.

Deglaze the pan, and whisk the cream sauce. Toss in the greens until thoroughly coated with the sauce.

Arrange the thighs on the greens, warm up, and serve.

Nutrition:

Calories: 446

Net Carbs: 3 g

Total Fat Content: 38 g

Protein: 18 g

Curry Chicken Lettuce Wraps

Preparation Time: 15 minutes

Cooking Time: 10 minutes
Servings: 5
Ingredients:
2 Minced garlic cloves
.25 cups Minced onion
1 lb. Chicken thighs – skinless & boneless
2 tbsp. Ghee
1 tsp. Black pepper
2 tsp. Curry powder
1.5 tsp. Salt
1 cup Riced cauliflower
5-6 Lettuce leaves
Keto-friendly sour cream (as desired - count the carbs)
Directions:
Mince the garlic and onions. Set aside for now.
Pull out the bones and skin from the chicken and dice into one-inch pieces.
On the stovetop, add 2 tbsp. of ghee to a skillet and melt. Toss in the onion and sauté until browned. Fold in the chicken and sprinkle with the garlic, pepper, and salt.
Cook for eight minutes. Stir in the remainder of the ghee, riced cauliflower, and curry. Stir until well mixed.
Prepare the lettuce leaves and add the mixture.
Serve with a dollop of cream.
Nutrition:
Calories: 554
Net Carbs: 7 g
Total Fat Content: 36 g
Protein: 50 g

Nacho Chicken Casserole

Preparation Time: 15 minutes
Cooking Time: 25 minutes
Servings: 6
Ingredients:
1 medium Jalapeño pepper
1.75 lb. Chicken thighs
Pepper and salt (to taste)
2 tbsp. Olive oil
1.5 tsp. Chili seasoning
4 oz. Cheddar cheese
4 oz. Cream cheese
3 tbsp. Parmesan cheese
1 cup Green chilies and tomatoes
.25 cup Sour cream

1 pkg. Frozen cauliflower
Also Needed: Immersion blender
Directions:
Warm the oven to reach 375º Fahrenheit.
Slice the jalapeño into pieces and set aside.
Cutaway the skin and bones from the chicken. Chop it and sprinkle using the pepper and salt. Prepare in a skillet using a portion of olive oil on the med-high temperature setting until browned.
Mix in the sour cream, cream cheese, and ¾ of the cheddar cheese. Stir until melted and combined well. Place in the tomatoes and chilies. Stir then put it all to a baking dish.
Cook the cauliflower in the microwave. Blend in the rest of the cheese with the immersion blender until it resembles mashed potatoes. Season as desired.
Spread the cauliflower concoction over the casserole and sprinkle with the peppers. Bake approximately 15 to 20 minutes.
Nutrition:
Calories: 426
Net Carbs: 4.3 g
Total Fat Content: 32.2 g
Protein: 31 g

Pesto & Mozzarella Chicken Casserole

Preparation Time: 10 minutes
Cooking Time: 25-30 minutes
Servings: 8
Ingredients:
Cooking oil (as needed)
2 lb. Grilled & cubed chicken breasts
8 oz. Cubed mozzarella
8 oz. Cream cheese
8 oz. Shredded mozzarella
.25 cup Pesto
.25 to .5 cup Heavy cream
Directions:
Warm the oven to 400º Fahrenheit. Spritz a casserole dish with a spritz of cooking oil spray.
Combine the pesto, heavy cream, and softened cream cheese.
Add the chicken and cubed mozzarella into the greased dish.
Sprinkle the chicken using the shredded mozzarella. Bake for 25-30 minutes.
Nutrition:
Calories: 451
Net Carbs: 3 g
Total Fat Content: 30 g
Protein: 38 g

Rotisserie Chicken & Cabbage Shreds

Preparation Time: 10 minutes
Cooking Time: 0 minutes
Servings: 2
Ingredients:
.5 of 1 Red onion
7 oz. Fresh green cabbage
1 lb. Precooked rotisserie chicken
.5 cup Keto-friendly mayo
1 tbsp. Olive oil
Pepper & Salt
Direction:
Use a sharp kitchen knife to shred the cabbage and slice the onion into thin slices.
Place the chicken on a platter, add the mayo, and a drizzle of oil. Dust using salt and pepper.
Serve.
Nutrition:
Calories: 423
Net Carbs: 6 g
Total Fat Content: 35 g
Protein: 17 g

Chicken Quiche

Preparation Time: 15 minutes
Cooking Time: 50 minutes
Servings: 6
Ingredients:
16 oz. almond flour
7 medium eggs
Salt and ground black pepper to taste
2 tbsp. coconut oil
1 lb. ground chicken
2 small zucchini, grated
1 tsp dried oregano
1 tsp fennel seeds
½ cup heavy cream
Directions:
Place almond flour, 1 egg, salt, and coconut oil in blender or food processor and blend.
Grease pie pan and pour the dough in it. Press well on the bottom.
Preheat pan on medium heat and toss ground chicken, cook for 2 minutes, set aside.
In a medium bowl, whisk together 6 eggs, zucchini, oregano, salt, pepper, fennel seeds, and heavy cream.
Add chicken to egg mixture and stir well.
Preheat oven to 350 F.

Pour egg mixture into pie pan and place in oven. Cook for 40 minutes.
Let it cool and slice. Serve.
Nutrition:
Calories
295
Carbs 3.95g
Fat 24g
Protein 19g

Chicken Parmigiana

Preparation Time: 15 minutes
Cooking Time: 26 minutes
Servings: 4
Ingredients:
1 large organic egg, beaten
½ cup of superfine blanched almond flour
¼ cup Parmesan cheese, grated
½ teaspoon dried parsley
½ teaspoon paprika
½ teaspoon garlic powder
Salt and ground black pepper, as required
4 -6-ounces grass-fed skinless, boneless chicken breasts, pounded into a ½-inch thickness
¼ cup olive oil
1½ cups marinara sauce
4 ounces mozzarella cheese, thinly sliced
2 tablespoons fresh parsley, chopped
Directions:
Preheat the oven to 375 degrees F.
Add the beaten egg into a shallow dish.
Place the almond flour, Parmesan, parsley, spices, salt, and black pepper in another shallow dish and mix well.
Dip each chicken breast into the beaten egg and then coat with the flour mixture.
Heat the oil in a deep skillet over medium-high heat and fry the chicken breasts for about 3 minutes per side.
Using a slotted spoon, moved the chicken breasts onto a paper towel-lined plate to drain.
At the bottom of a casserole, put about ½ cup of marinara sauce and spread evenly.
Arrange the chicken breasts over marinara sauce in a single layer.
Top with the remaining marinara sauce, followed by mozzarella cheese slices.
Bake for about at least 20 minutes or until done completely.
Take off from the oven and serve hot with the garnishing of fresh parsley.
Nutrition:
Calories: 542
Net Carbs: 5.7g

Carbohydrate: 9g
Fiber: 3.3g
Protein: 54.2g
Fat: 33.2g
Sugar: 3.8g
Sodium: 609mg

Vegetarian Ketogenic Burgers

Preparation Time: 10 minutes
Cooking Time: 10 minutes
Servings: 2
Ingredients:
1 garlic cloves, minced
2 Portobello mushrooms
1 tbsp. coconut oil, melted
1 tbsp. chopped basil
1 tbsp. oregano
2 eggs, fried
2 zero carb buns
2 tbsp. mayonnaise
2 lettuce leaves
Salt to taste
Directions:
Combine the coconut oil, garlic, basil, oregano, and salt in a bowl. Place the mushrooms in the bowl and coat well. Preheat the grill to medium. Grill the mushrooms about 2 minutes per side. Slice them and grill for 2 minutes per side. Cut the buns in half. Add the lettuce leaves, mushrooms, eggs, and mayo. Top with the other bun.
Nutrition:
Calories 637;
Net Carbs 8.5g
Fat 53g
Protein 23g

Tempeh Taco Cups

Preparation Time: 10 minutes
Cooking Time: 25 minutes
Servings: 4
Ingredients:
8 iceberg lettuce leaves
4 zero carb tortilla wraps
2 tsp melted butter
1 tbsp. olive oil
1 yellow onion, chopped
½ cup tempeh, crumbled

1 tsp smoked paprika
½ tsp cumin powder
1 red bell pepper, chopped
1 avocado, halved and pitted
1 small lemon, juiced
¼ cup sour cream
Directions:
Preheat oven to 400 F. Divide each tortilla wrap into 2, lay on a chopping board, and brush with butter. Line 8 muffin tins with the tortilla and bake for 9 minutes.
Heat olive oil in a skillet and sauté onion for 3 minutes. Crumble tempeh into the pan and cook for 8 minutes. Stir in paprika and cumin and cook for 1 minute. To assemble, fit lettuce leaves into the tortilla cups, share tempeh mixture on top, top with bell pepper, avocado, and drizzle with lemon juice. Add sour cream and serve.
Nutrition:
Calories 220
Net Carbs 3.8g
Fat 17g
Protein 6.7g

Mushroom White Pizza

Preparation Time: 10 minutes
Cooking Time: 25 minutes
Servings: 4
Ingredients:
2 eggs
½ cup mayonnaise
¾ cup almond flour
1 tbsp. psyllium husk powder
1 tsp baking soda
½ tsp salt
¼ cup mushrooms, sliced
1 tbsp. oregano
1 tbsp. basil pesto
2 tbsp. olive oil
Salt and black pepper to taste
½ cup coconut cream
¾ cup Parmesan, shredded
6 black olives
Directions:
In a bowl, whisk eggs and mix in mayonnaise, almond flour, psyllium husk powder, baking soda, and salt. Allow sitting for 5 minutes. Pour the batter into a greased baking sheet. Bake for 10 minutes at 350 F. In a bowl, mix mushrooms with pesto, olive oil, salt, and pepper. Take off the crust from the oven and spread the coconut cream on top. Add the mushroom

mixture and Parmesan cheese. Bake the pizza further until the cheese melts, about 10 minutes. Spread the olives on top and serve.

Nutrition:
Calories 346
Net Carbs 5.5g
Fat 32.7g
Protein 8g

Cheesy Broccoli Nachos with Salsa

Preparation Time: 5 minutes
Cooking Time: 20 minutes
Servings: 4

Ingredients:
2 heads broccoli, chopped
3 tbsp. coconut flour
1 tsp smoked paprika
½ tsp coriander powder
1 tsp cumin powder
½ tsp garlic powder
2 eggs, beaten
¼ cup grated Monterey Jack
4 plum tomatoes, chopped
½ lime, juiced
4 sprigs cilantro, chopped
1 avocado, chopped

Directions:
Preheat oven to 350 F. Pour broccoli in a food processor and blend into a rice-like consistency. Heat a skillet over low heat, pour in broccoli, and fry for 10 minutes. Transfer to a bowl. Line 2 baking sheets with parchment papers. To the broccoli, add coconut flour, paprika, coriander powder, cumin, garlic, and eggs. Mix and form into a ball. Divide into halves, place each half on each baking sheet, and press down into a rough circle. Bake for 10 minutes. Take it out from the oven, cut into triangles, and sprinkle with Monterey Jack cheese; let cool. In a bowl, combine tomatoes, lime, cilantro, and avocado. Serve nachos with salsa.

Nutrition:
Calories 208
Net Carbs 4.5g
Fat 12.4g
Protein 7g

One-Skillet Green Pasta

Preparation Time: 10 minutes
Cooking Time: 5 minutes
Servings: 4

Ingredients:
1 cup shredded mozzarella cheese
1 cup grated Pecorino Romano cheese for topping
1 egg yolk
2 garlic cloves, minced
1 lemon, juiced
1 cup baby spinach
½ cup almond milk
1 avocado, pitted and peeled
1 tbsp. olive oil
Salt to taste
Directions:
Microwave mozzarella cheese for 2 minutes. Take out the bowl and allow cooling for 1 minute. Mix in egg yolk until well-combined. Lay a parchment paper on a flat surface, pour the cheese mixture on top, and cover it with another parchment paper. Flatten the dough into 1/8-inch thickness. Take off the parchment paper and cut the dough into thick fettuccine strands. Place in a bowl and refrigerate overnight. Place 2 cups water to a boil in a saucepan and add the fettuccine. Cook for 1 minute and drain; set aside. In a blender, combine garlic, lemon juice, spinach, almond milk, avocado, olive oil, and salt. Process until smooth. Pour fettuccine into a bowl, top with sauce, and mix. Top with Pecorino Romano cheese and serve.
Nutrition:
Calories 290
Net Carbs 5g
Fats 19g
Protein 18g

Charred Asparagus with Creamy Sauce

Preparation Time: 5 minutes
Cooking Time: 7 minutes
Servings: 4
Ingredients:
½ lb. asparagus, no hard stalks
Salt and chili pepper to taste
4 tbsp. flax seed powder
½ cup coconut cream
1 cup butter, melted
⅓ cup mozzarella, grated
2 tbsp. olive oil
Juice of half lemon
Directions:
Warm olive oil in a saucepan then roast the asparagus until lightly charred. Season with salt and set aside. Melt half of butter in a pan and stir until nutty and golden brown. Add in

lemon juice and pour the mixture over the asparagus. In a safe microwave bowl, mix flax seed powder with ½ cup water and let sit for 5 minutes. Microwave flax egg 1-2 minutes, then pour into a blender. Add the remaining butter, mozzarella cheese, coconut cream, salt, and chili pepper. Puree until well combined and smooth. Serve.

Nutrition:

Calories 442

Net Carbs 5.4g

Fat 45g

Protein 5.9g

Mozzarella Fish

Preparation Time: 5 minutes

Cooking Time: 10-15 minutes

Servings: 6-8

Ingredients:

2 lbs. of bone gold sole

Salt and pepper to taste

½ teaspoon dried oregano

1 cup grated mozzarella cheese

1 large fresh tomato, sliced thinly

Directions:

Excellent source of cooking the butter. Organize a single layer of trout. Add salt, pepper, and oregano.

Top with sliced cheese slices and tomatoes.

Cook, covered, for 10 to 15 minutes at 425°F.

Nutrition:

Calories: 156

Fat: 6g

Net Carbs: 5g

Protein: 8g

Cheesy Bacon-Wrapped Chicken with Asparagus Spears

Preparation Time: 20 minutes

Cooking Time: 30 minutes

Servings: 4

Ingredients:

4 chicken breasts

8 bacon slices

1 pound (454 g) asparagus spears

2 tablespoons fresh lemon juice

½ cup Manchego cheese, grated

From the cupboard

4 tablespoons olive oil, divided

Salt, to taste

Freshly ground black pepper, to taste
Directions:
Set the oven to 400ºF. Line a baking sheet using parchment paper, then grease with 1 tablespoon olive oil.
Put the chicken breasts in a large bowl, and sprinkle with salt and black pepper. Toss to combine well.
Wrap every chicken breast with 2 slices of bacon. Place the chicken on the baking sheet, then bake in the preheated oven for 25 minutes or until the bacon is crispy.
Preheat the grill to high, then brush with the remaining olive oil.
Place the asparagus spears on the grill grate, and sprinkle with salt. Grill for 5 minutes or until fork-tender. Flip the asparagus frequently during the grilling.
Transfer the bacon-wrapped chicken breasts to four plates, drizzle with lemon juice, and scatter with Manchego cheese. Spread the hot asparagus spears on top to serve.
Nutrition:
Calories: 455
Total fat: 38.1g
Net carbs: 2g
Protein: 26.1g

Bacon-Wrapped Chicken with Cheddar Cheese

Preparation Time: 10 minutes
Cooking Time:
4 hours
Servings: 6
Ingredients:
2 large chicken breasts, each cut into 6 pieces
6 slices of streaky bacon, each cut in half widthways
4 garlic cloves, crushed
½ cup Cheddar cheese, grated
From the cupboard:
1 tablespoon olive oil
Salt, to taste
Freshly ground black pepper, to taste
Directions:
Grease the insert of the slow cooker with olive oil.
Wrap each piece of chicken breast with each half of the bacon slice, and arrange them in the slow cooker. Sprinkle with garlic, salt, and black pepper.
Put the lid and then cook on LOW for 4 hours.
Set the oven to 350ºF (180ºC).
Transfer the cooked bacon-wrapped chicken to a baking dish, then scatter with cheese.
Cook in the preheated oven for 5 minutes or until the cheese melts.
Take it off from the oven and serve warm.
Nutrition:

Calories: 308
Total fat: 20.8g
Total carbs: 2.9g
Fiber: 0g
Net carbs: 2.9g
Protein: 26.1g

Delightful Teriyaki Chicken Under Pressure

Preparation Time: 5 minutes
Cooking Time: 20 minutes
Servings: 8
Ingredients:
1 cup Chicken Broth
¾ cup Brown Sugar
2 tbsp. ground Ginger
1 tsp Pepper
3 pounds Boneless and Skinless Chicken Thighs
¼ cup Apple Cider Vinegar
¾ cup low-sodium Soy Sauce
20 ounces canned Pineapple, crushed
2 tbsp. Garlic Powder
Directions:
Mix all of the ingredients, excluding the chicken. Add the chicken meat and turn to coat. Seal the lid, press POULTRY, and cook for 20 minutes at High. Do a quick pressure release by turning the valve to an "open" position.
Nutrition:
Calories 352
Carbs 31g
Fat 11g
Protein 31g

Turkey and Potatoes with Buffalo Sauce

Preparation Time: 10 minutes
Cooking Time: 20 minutes
Servings: 2
Ingredients:
3 tbsps. Olive Oil
4 tbsp. Buffalo Sauce
1 pound Sweet Potatoes, cut into cubes
1 ½ pound Turkey Breast, cut into pieces
½ tsp Garlic Powder
1 Onion, diced
½ cup Water
Directions:

Heat 1 tbsp. Of olive oil on SAUTÉ mode at High. Stir-fry onion in hot oil for about 3 minutes. Stir in the remaining ingredients. Seal the lid, set to PRESSURE COOK/MANUAL mode for 20 minutes at high pressure.
When cooking is over, do a quick pressure release by turning the valve to an "open" position. Nutrition:
Calories 377
Carbs 32g
Fat 9g
Protein 14g

Happy Burrito Bowl Pork

Preparation Time: 10 minutes
Cooking Time: 5 minutes
Servings: 4
Ingredients:
1 and ½ tablespoons pork lard
1 onion, sliced
2 bell peppers, sliced
1 garlic clove, chopped
Salt and pepper to taste
1 pound pulled pork
½ cup of chicken pork
½ cup chicken broth
6 cups lettuce, chopped
6 cups cabbage, chopped
¼ cup guacamole
Directions:
Set your Ninja Foodi to Saute mode and add lard, let it melt and add onion and bell pepper
Cook for 2 minutes, stirring for 2 minutes. Add garlic, salt, and pepper
Stir well. Add pulled pork and chicken pork
Lock lid and cook on high pressure for 1 minute. Quick-release pressure
Arrange lettuce and green cabbage in serving bowls and add pulled pork on top
Top with guacamole and serve. Enjoy!
Nutrition:
Calories: 417
Fat: 95g
Carbohydrates: 6g
Protein: 75g

Sauerkraut Pork

Preparation Time: 10 minutes
Cooking Time: 35 minutes
Servings: 4
Ingredients:

3 pounds of pork shoulder
Salt and pepper to taste
3 tablespoons butter
2 onions, chopped
3 cloves garlic, sliced
6 cups sauerkraut, divided
1-pound hot dog, sliced and cooked
½ pound kielbasa, sliced and cooked
Directions:
Season pork roast with salt and pepper
Set your Ninja Foodi to Sauté mode and add butter, let the butter melt
Add pork roast and brown. Pour 2 cups water, onion and garlic
Season with salt and pepper and lock lid. Cook on high pressure for 35 minutes
Release pressure naturally over 10 minutes
Shred pork and stir in sauerkraut, hotdog, and kielbasa. Serve and enjoy!
Nutrition:
Calories: 792
Fat: 83g
Carbohydrates: 14g
Protein: 68g

Jalapeno Hash

Preparation Time: 5 minutes
Cooking Time: 10 minutes
Servings: 4
Ingredients:
4 jalapeno peppers, chopped
½ cup chicken stock
3 ounces bacon, chopped and cooked
6 ounces zucchini, chopped
1 teaspoon ground black pepper
1 teaspoon butter
Directions:
Add jalapeno peppers and zucchini into the Ninja Foodi pot
Put bacon, ground black pepper, butter, and chicken stock
Seal the lid. Set Pressure High. Cook the meat for 5 minutes
Then make natural pressure release for 10 minutes
Once cooked, let the meal chill for a few minutes. Serve with chicken stock and enjoy!
Nutrition:
Calories: 139
Fat: 10.3g
Carbohydrates: 3.2g
Protein: 8.8g

The Premium Red Pork

Preparation Time: 10 minutes
Cooking Time: 40 minutes
Servings: 6
Ingredients:
2 pounds of pork belly
2 tablespoons maple syrup
3 tablespoons sherry
1 tablespoon blackstrap molasses
2 tablespoons coconut amino
1 teaspoon salt
1/3 cup water
1-piece ginger, peeled and smashed
Few sprigs of cilantro, garnish
Directions:
Add the pork cubes to a pot and place it over medium heat
Add enough water to submerge them. Let the water boil.
Boil the cubes for 3 minutes and drain and rinse the cubes to remove any impurities
Keep them on the side. Set your Ninja Foodi to Saute mode and add maple syrup
Add cooked cubes and cook them for 1 minute until browned
After 10 minutes, add the remaining ingredients into the mix and bring the whole mixture to a boil. Lock up the lid and cook for 25 minutes at high pressure
Allow the pressure to release naturally.
Open up the lid and set your Ninja Foodi to Saute mode again
Let the content it simmer for a while until the liquid has been reduced sufficiently to coat the cubes. Serve with a garnish of cilantro. Enjoy!
Nutrition:
Calories: 335
Fats: 13g
Carbohydrates:16g
Protein:31g

Spicy Pork Salad Bowl

Preparation Time: 10 minutes
Cooking Time: 90 minutes
Servings: 6
Ingredients:
4 pounds pork shoulder butter
2 teaspoons salt
2 cups chicken stock
1 teaspoon smoked paprika powder
1 teaspoon garlic powder
1 teaspoon black pepper

1 pinch dried oregano leaves
4 tablespoons coconut oil
6 garlic cloves
Directions
Remove rind from pork and cut meat from the bone, slice into large chunks
Trim fat off met
Set your Foodi to Saute mode and add oil, let it heat up
Once the oil is hot, layer chunks of meat in the bottom of the pot and Saute for around 30 minutes until browned
While the meat is being browned, peel garlic cloves and cut into small chunks
When the meat is browned, take it to a large-sized bowl
Add a few tablespoons of chicken stock to the pot a deglaze it, scraping off browned bits
Transfer browned bits to the bowl with meat chunks. Repeat if any more meat is left
Once done, add garlic, oregano leaves, smoked paprika, Garlic powder, pepper, and salt to the meat owl and mix it up. Add all chicken stock to the pot and bring to a simmer over Saute mode
Once done, return seasoned meat to the pot and lock lid, cook on high pressure for 45 minutes. Release pressure naturally over 10 minutes
Open the lid and shred the meat using a fork, transfer shredded meat to a bowl and pour cooking liquid through a mesh to separate fat into the bowl with shredded meat
Serve with lime and enjoy!
Nutrition:
Calories: 307
Fat: 23g
Carbohydrates: 8g
Protein: 15g

Dill and Butter Pork Chops

Preparation Time: 10 minutes
Cooking Time: 20 minutes
Servings: 4
Ingredients:
2 tablespoons unsalted butter
4 pieces ½ inch thick pork loin chops
½ teaspoon salt
½ teaspoon pepper
16 baby carrots
½ cup white wine vinegar
½ cup chicken broth
Directions:
Set your Ninja Foodi to Saute mode. Season the chops with pepper and salt
Toss your chops into your pot and cook for 4 minutes
Transfer the chops to a plate and repeat to cook and brown the rest

Pour in 1 tablespoon of butter and Toss in your carrots, dill to the cooker and let it cook for about 1 minute

Put the wine and scrape off any browned bits in your cooker while the liquid comes to a boil

Stir in the broth. return the chops to your pot

Lock up the lid and let it cook for about 18 minutes at high pressure

Naturally, release the pressure by keeping it aside for 8 minutes

Unlock and serve with some sauce poured over

Nutrition:

Calories: 296

Fat: 25g

Carbohydrates: 2g

Protein: 17g

Cranberry Pork BBQ Dish

Preparation Time: 10 minutes

Cooking Time: 45 minutes

Servings: 4

Ingredients:

3-4 pounds pork shoulder, boneless, fat trimmed

For Sauce

3 tablespoons of liquid smoke

2 tablespoons tomato paste

2 cups fresh cranberries

¼ cup hot sauce

1/3 cup blackstrap molasses

½ cup of water

½ cup apple cider vinegar

1 teaspoon salt

1 tablespoon adobo sauce

1 cup tomato puree

1 chipotle pepper in adobo sauce, diced

Directions:

Cut pork against halves/thirds and keep it on the side

Set your Ninja Foodi to sauté mode and let it heat up. Add cranberries and water to the pot

Let them simmer for 4-5 minutes until cranberries start to pop, add rest of the sauce ingredients and simmer for 5 minutes more. Add pork to the pot and lock lid

Cook on high pressure for 40 minutes. Quick-release pressure

Use a fork to shred the pork and serve on your favorite greens

Nutrition:

Calories: 250

Fat: 17g

Carbohydrates: 5g

Protein: 15g

Pasta Orecchiette with Broccoli & Tofu

Preparation Time: 10 minutes
Cooking Time: 15 minutes
Servings: 4
Ingredients:
1 (9 oz.) pack orecchiette
16 oz. broccoli, roughly chopped
2 garlic cloves
3 tbsp. olive oil
1 tbsp. grated tofu
Salt and black pepper to taste
Directions:
Place the orecchiette and broccoli in your instant pot. Cover with water and seal the lid. Cook on High Pressure for 10 minutes. Do a quick release.
Drain the broccoli and orecchiette. Set aside. Heat the olive oil on Sauté mode. Stir-fry garlic for 2 minutes. Stir in broccoli, orecchiette, salt, and pepper. Cook for 2 more minutes. Press Cancel and Stir in grated tofu, to serve.
Nutrition:
Calories: 192 kcal
Protein: 7.08 g
Fat: 12.6 g
Carbohydrates: 16.93 g

Herbed Portobello Mushrooms

Preparation Time: 10 minutes
Cooking Time: 10 minutes
Servings: 2
Ingredients:
2 Portobello mushrooms, stemmed and wiped clean
1 tsp minced garlic
¼ tsp dried rosemary
1 tablespoon balsamic vinegar
¼ cup grated provolone cheese
4 tablespoons olive oil
Salt and pepper to taste
Directions:
In an oven, position rack 4-inches away from the top and preheat broiler.
Prepare a baking dish by spraying using cooking spray lightly.
Stemless, place mushroom gill side up.
Mix well garlic, rosemary, balsamic vinegar, and olive oil in a small bowl. Season with salt and pepper to taste.
Drizzle over mushrooms equally.

Marinate for at least 5 minutes before popping into the oven and broiling for 4 minutes per side or until tender.
Once cooked, remove from oven, sprinkle cheese, return to broiler and broil for a minute or two or until cheese melts.
Remove from oven and serve right away.
Nutrition:
Calories: 168
Fat: 5.1g
Carbs: 21.5g
Protein: 8.6g

Garlic ‘n Sour Cream Zucchini Bake

Preparation Time: 10 minutes
Cooking Time: 35 minutes
Servings: 3
Ingredients:
1 ½ cups zucchini slices
5 tablespoons olive oil
1 tablespoon minced garlic
1/4 cup grated Parmesan cheese
1 (8 ounces) package cream cheese, softened
Salt and pepper to taste
Directions:
Lightly grease a baking sheet using cooking spray.
Place zucchini in a bowl and put in olive oil and garlic.
Place zucchini slices in a single layer in dish.
Bake for 35 minutes at 390oF until crispy.
In a bowl, whisk well, remaining ingredients.
Serve with zucchini
Nutrition:
Calories: 385
Fat: 32.4g
Carbs: 9.5g
Protein: 11.9g

Paprika ‘n Cajun Seasoned Onion Rings

Preparation Time: 15 minutes
Cooking Time: 25 minutes
Servings: 6
Ingredients:
1 large white onion
2 large eggs, beaten
½ teaspoon Cajun seasoning
¾ cup almond flour

1 ½ teaspoon paprika
½ cups coconut oil for frying
¼ cup water
Salt and pepper to taste
Directions:
Preheat a pot with oil for 8 minutes.
Peel the onion cut off the top and slice into circles.
In a mixing bowl, combine the water and the eggs. Season with pepper and salt.
Soak the onion in the egg mixture.
In another bowl, combine the almond flour, paprika powder, Cajun seasoning, salt, and pepper.
Dredge the onion in the almond flour mixture.
Place in the pot and cook in batches until golden brown, around 8 minutes per batch.
Nutrition:
Calories: 262
Fat: 24.1g
Carbs: 3.9g
Protein: 2.8g

Grilled Parmesan Eggplant

Preparation Time: 5 minutes
Cooking Time: 15 minutes
Servings: 4
Ingredients:
1 medium-sized eggplant
1 log (1 lb.) fresh mozzarella cheese, cut into sixteen
1 small tomato, cut into eight slices
1/2 cup shredded Parmesan cheese
Chopped fresh basil or parsley
1/2 teaspoon salt
1 tablespoon olive oil
1/2 teaspoon pepper
Directions:
Trim ends of the eggplant; cut eggplant crosswise into eight slices. Dust with salt; let stand 5 minutes.
Blot eggplant dry with paper towels; brush each side with oil and sprinkle with pepper. Grill, covered, over medium heat 4-6 minutes on each side or until tender. Remove from grill.
Top eggplant with mozzarella cheese, tomato, and Parmesan cheese. Grill, covered, 1-2 minutes longer or until cheese begins to melt. Top with basil.
Nutrition:
Calories: 449
Fat: 31g

Carbs: 10g
Protein: 26g

Exquisite Pear and Onion Goose

Preparation Time: 15 minutes
Cooking Time: 20 minutes
Servings: 8
Ingredients:
2 cups Chicken Broth
1 tbsp. Butter
½ cup slice Onions
1 ½ pounds Goose, chopped into large pieces
2 tbsp. Balsamic Vinegar
1 tsp Cayenne Pepper
3 Pears, peeled and sliced
¼ tsp Garlic Powder
½ tsp Pepper
Directions:
Melt the butter on SAUTÉ. Add the goose and cook until it becomes golden on all sides. Transfer to a plate. Add the onions and cook for 2 minutes. Return the goose to the cooker. Add the rest of the ingredients, stir well to combine and seal the lid. Select PRESSURE COOK/MANUAL mode, and set the timer to 18 minutes at High Pressure. Do a quick pressure release. Serve and enjoy!
Nutrition:
Calories 313
Carbs 14g
Fat 8g
Protein 38g

Turkey Breast with Fennel and Celery

Preparation Time: 10 minutes
Cooking Time: 15 minutes
Servings: 3
Ingredients:
2 pounds Boneless and Skinless Turkey Breast
1 cup Fennel Bulb, chopped
1 cup celery with leaves, chopped
2 ¼ cups Chicken Stock
¼ tsp Pepper
¼ tsp Garlic Powder
Directions:
Throw all ingredients in your pressure cooker. Give it a good stir and seal the lid. Press PRESSURE COOK/MANUAL, and cook for 15 minutes at High. Do a quick pressure release. Shred the turkey with two forks.

Nutrition:
Calories 272
Carbs 7g
Fat 4g
Protein 48g

Pancetta and Chicken Risotto

Preparation Time: 15 minutes
Cooking Time: 15 minutes
Servings: 2
Ingredients:
3/4-pound. Chicken meat, diced
2 to 3 slices pancetta; diced
3/4 cup risotto or Arborio rice
1 teaspoon fresh thyme
1 tablespoon lemon zest
1 tablespoon unsalted butter
1 tablespoon olive oil
2 tablespoon parmesan; grated
2 garlic cloves; chopped
1/2 onion; chopped
1/3 cup white wine
3 ½ cups chicken stock
Salt and Pepper to taste
Directions:
Put oil and butter to Instant Pot and press the "Sauté" button (*Normal* preset), wait till you see Hot on display.
Add onion, cook for 1 to 2 minutes. Add pancetta, chicken, and garlic. Cook for another 2 to 3 minutes.
Add rice and mix well, the rice should be covered with oil-butter mixture. Pour the wine and scrape the sides of the pot. Cook for 2 to 3 minutes, stirring constantly. Press *Cancel* button.
Add chicken stock, thyme, lemon zest, salt, and pepper. Seal the lid and turn the vent to *Sealed*. Press *Pressure Cook* (Manual) button, use *+* or *-* button to set the timer for 6 minutes. Use *Pressure level* button to set Pressure to *HIGH*.
When the timer is up, press *Cancel* button and allow the pressure to be released naturally; until the float valve drops down.
Open the lid; Add parmesan cheese to the pot and stir well until it melts. Serve topped with extra parmesan and lemon zest.
Nutrition:
Calories: 586 g
Total Fat: 22.5 g
Total Carbohydrate: 23.6 g

Protein: 45

Popcorn Shrimp

Preparation Time: 5 minutes
Cooking Time: 20 minutes
Servings: 2
Ingredients:
1/2 lb. (225 g) small shrimp, peeled
2 eggs, whisked
6 Tablespoons (36 g) cajun seasoning
6 Tablespoons (42 g) coconut flour
Coconut oil for frying
Directions:
Warm the coconut oil in a saucepan (use enough coconut oil so that it's 1/2 inch (1-2 cm) deep) or deep fryer.
Place the whisked eggs into a large bowl, and in another large bowl, combine the coconut flour and seasoning.
Toss a handful of the shrimp into the whisked eggs and stir around so that each shrimp is coated.
Then take the shrimp out of the whisked eggs the put into the seasoning bowl. Coat the shrimp using the coconut flour and seasoning mixture.
Bring the coated shrimp into the hot oil and fry until golden. (Don't stir the pot and the shrimp must in deep-fried)
Using a slotted spoon, take off the shrimp and place on paper towels to absorb the excess oil. Repeat for the remaining shrimp (change the oil if there are too many solids in it).
Cool for at least 10 minutes.
Nutrition:
Calories: 390
Fat: 23 g
Net Carbohydrates: 3 g
Protein: 30 g

Cucumber Ginger Shrimp

Preparation Time: 5 minutes
Cooking Time: 10 minutes
Servings: 1
Ingredients:
1 large cucumber, sliced into 1/2-inch round
10-15 large shrimp/prawns
1 teaspoon (1 g) fresh ginger, grated
Salt to taste
Coconut oil to cook with
Directions:
Pour 1 Tablespoon (15 ml) of coconut oil into a frying pan on medium heat.

Put the ginger and the cucumber and sauté for 2-3 minutes.
Add in the shrimp then cook until they turn pink and are no longer translucent.
Add salt to taste and serve.
Nutrition:
Calories: 250
Fat: 16 g
Net Carbohydrates: 4 g
Protein: 20 g

Salmon with Pesto

Preparation Time: 10 minutes
Cooking Time: 15 minutes
Servings: 4
Ingredients:
4 salmon fillets
2 teaspoons olive oil
Pinch of salt
½-cup pesto
Directions:
Arrange the greased Cook & Crisp Basket in the pot of Ninja Foodi.
Close the Ninja Foodi with crisping lid and select Air Crisp.
Set the temperature to 270 degrees F for 5 minutes.
Press Start/Stop to begin preheating.
Drizzle the salmon fillets with oil evenly and sprinkle with a pinch of salt.
After preheating, open the lid.
Place the salmon fillets into the Cook & Crisp Basket.
Close the Ninja Foodi with crisping lid and select Air Crisp.
Set the temperature to 270 degrees F for 20 minutes.
Press Start/Stop to begin cooking.
Transfer the salmon fillets onto a platter and top with the pesto.
Serve immediately.
Nutrition:
Calories: 380
Fats: 25.8g
Carbohydrates: 2g
Proteins: 36g

Salmon in Dill Sauce

Preparation Time: 10 minutes
Cooking Time: 2 hours
Servings: 6
Ingredients:
2 cups water
1-cup homemade chicken broth

2 tablespoons fresh lemon juice
¼ cup fresh dill, chopped
6 salmon fillets
1 teaspoon cayenne pepper
Salt and ground black pepper
Directions:
In the pot of Ninja Foodi, mix together the water, broth, lemon juice, lemon juice and dill.
Organize the salmon fillets on top, skin side down, and sprinkle with cayenne pepper, salt black pepper.
Close the Ninja Foodi with crisping lid and select Slow Cooker.
Set on Low for 1-2 hours.
Press Start/Stop to begin cooking.
Serve hot.
Nutrition:
Calories: 164
Fats: 7.4g
Carbohydrates 1.6 g
Proteins: 23.3g

Flay Beef Empanadas

Preparation Time: 30 minutes
Cooking Time: 25 minutes
Servings: 6
Ingredients:
For the Dough
1 cup mozzarella cheese, shredded
5 tablespoons cream cheese
¾ cup almond flour
2 tablespoons coconut milk
1 tablespoon coconut flour
1 egg, lightly beaten
1 teaspoon garlic powder
½ teaspoon sea salt
Directions:
To make the Dough:
Melt the cheeses. In a small pan at low heat, melt the mozzarella and cream cheese together, stirring often. Remove the pan from the heat.
Mix the dough. Transfer the cheese mixture to a medium bowl and stir in the almond flour, coconut milk, coconut flour, egg, garlic powder, and salt until everything is well blended and the mixture holds together in a ball. Cover the bowl using plastic wrap, pressing it down onto the surface of the dough, and place the bowl in the refrigerator for 30 minutes.
For the Filling:
¼ cup grass-fed butter

1 pound grass-fed ground beef
1 onion, chopped
1 tablespoon minced garlic
2 tablespoons sugar-free tomato paste
2 teaspoons ground cumin
2 teaspoons dried oregano
1 teaspoon chili powder
Sea salt, for seasoning
Freshly ground black pepper, for seasoning
Directions:
To make the Filling
Cook the beef. In a large skillet at medium-high heat, melt the butter. Put the beef and cook it until it's browned about 7 minutes.
Finish the filling. Add the onion and garlic and sauté until they've softened about 4 minutes. Stir in the tomato paste, cumin, oregano, and chili powder. Season the filling using pepper and salt, then set it aside to cool.
Directions:
To make Empanadas:
Preheat the oven. Set the oven temperature to 425°F. Line a baking sheet with parchment paper.
Cut the dough. Spread some parchment paper on your work surface. Press the dough out into a thin layer on the paper, and then cut the dough into 12 (3-inch) circles.
Fill the dough. Spoon the filling equally onto the middle of each dough circle. Fold the dough over, then press the sides together using a fork to seal them.
Bake. Transfer the empanadas to the baking sheet and bake them for 10 to 12 minutes until they are golden brown.
Serve. Divide the empanadas between six plates and serve them immediately.
Nutrition:
Calories: 436
Total fat: 38g
Total carbs: 4g
Fiber: 1g
Net carbs: 3g
Sodium: 229mg
Protein: 19g

Basil Halibut Red Pepper Packets

Preparation Time: 10 minutes
Cooking Time: 20 minutes
Servings: 4
Ingredients:
2 cups cauliflower florets
1 cup roasted red pepper strips

½ cup sliced sun-dried tomatoes
4 (4-ounce) halibut fillets
¼ cup chopped fresh basil
Juice of 1 lemon
¼ cup good-quality olive oil
Sea salt, for seasoning
Freshly ground black pepper, for seasoning
Directions:
Preheat the oven. Set the oven temperature to 400°F. Cut into four (12-inch) square pieces of aluminum foil. Have a baking sheet ready.
Make the packets. Divide the cauliflower, red pepper strips, and sun-dried tomato between the four pieces of foil, placing the vegetables in the middle of each piece. Top each pile with 1 halibut fillet, and top each fillet with equal amounts of the basil, lemon juice, and olive oil. Fold and crimp the foil to form sealed packets of fish and vegetables and place them on the baking sheet.
Bake. Bake the packets for about 20 minutes, until the fish flakes with a fork. Be careful of the steam when you open the packet!
Serve. Transfer the vegetables and halibut to four plates, season with salt and pepper, and serve immediately.
Nutrition:
Calories: 294
Total fat: 18g
Total carbs: 8g
Fiber: 3g
Net carbs: 5g
Sodium: 114mg
Protein: 25g

Bistecca Alla Florentina

Preparation Time: 10 minutes
Cooking Time: 15 minutes
Servings: 4
Ingredients:
2 (1-inch-thick) bone-in porterhouse steaks, about 2 pounds
6 tablespoons good-quality olive oil, divided
Sea salt, for seasoning
Freshly ground black pepper, for seasoning
½ cup white wine
2 rosemary sprigs
Lemon wedges, for serving
Directions:
Preheat the grill. Preheat the grill to high heat.

Prepare the steaks. Rub the steaks of 2 tbsp. of the olive oil and season them generously with salt and pepper.
Prepare the basting liquid. In a small bowl, stir together the white wine and the remaining 4 tablespoons of olive oil.
Grill the steaks. Using the rosemary sprigs as basters, baste the steaks on each side with the wine mixture. Grill the steaks, flipping them once until they are seared on both sides, 6 to 8 minutes in total (125°F internal temperature) for medium-rare.
Serve. Let the steaks rest for 10 minutes, divide them between four plates, and serve them with lemon wedges.
Nutrition:
Calories: 569
Total fat: 45g
Total carbs: 0g
Fiber: 0g
Net carbs: 0g
Sodium: 238mg
Protein: 35g

Zucchini Noodle Beef Lasagna

Preparation Time: 30 minutes
Cooking Time: 45minutes
Servings: 4
Ingredients:
2 tbsp. olive oil
½ red chili, chopped
1 lb. ground beef
3 large zucchinis, sliced lengthwise
2 garlic cloves, minced
1 shallot, chopped
1 cup tomato sauce
Salt and black pepper to taste
2 tsp sweet paprika
1 tsp dried thyme
1 tsp dried basil
1 cup mozzarella cheese, shredded
1 cup chicken broth
Directions:
Warm the oil in a skillet and then cook the beef for 4 minutes while breaking any lumps as you stir. Top with shallot, garlic, chili, tomatoes, salt, paprika, and black pepper. Stir and cook for 5 more minutes.
Lay 1/3 of the zucchinis slices in a greased baking dish. Top of 1/3 of the beef mixture and repeat the layering process twice with the same quantities. Season with basil and thyme. Pour in the chicken broth. Sprinkle the mozzarella cheese on top and tuck the baking dish

in the oven. Bake for 35 minutes at 380 F. Remove the lasagna and let it rest for 10 minutes before serving.
Nutrition:
Calories: 451
Fat 22.8g
Net Carbs 6.8g
Protein 42g

Chapter 3: Keto Dessert Recipes

Mocha Mousse

Preparation Time: 2 hours and 35 minutes
Cooking Time: 0
Servings: 4
Ingredients:
For the Cream Cheese:
Cream cheese, softened and full-fat - 8 ounces
Sour cream, full-fat - 3 tablespoons
Butter, softened - 2 tablespoons
Vanilla extract, unsweetened - 1 ½ teaspoons
Erythritol - 1/3 cup
Cocoa powder, unsweetened - ¼ cup
Instant coffee powder - 3 teaspoons
For the Whipped Cream:
Heavy whipping cream, full-fat - 2/3 cup
Erythritol - 1 ½ teaspoon
Vanilla extract, unsweetened - ½ teaspoon
Directions:
Prepare cream cheese mixture: For this, place cream cheese in a bowl, add sour cream and butter then beat until smooth.
Now add erythritol, cocoa powder, coffee, and vanilla and blend until incorporated, set aside until required.
Prepare whipping cream: For this, place whipping cream in a bowl and beat until soft peaks form.
Beat in vanilla and erythritol until stiff peaks form, then add 1/3 of the mixture into cream cheese mixture and fold until just mixed.
Then add remaining whipping cream mixture and fold until evenly incorporated.
Spoon the mousse into a freezer-proof bowl and place in the refrigerator for 2 ½ hours until set.
Serve straight away.
Nutrition:
Calories: 421.7;
Fat: 42 g;
Protein: 6 g;

Net Carbs: 6.5 g;
Fiber: 2 g;

Orange Custard Cups

Preparation Time: 4 hours and 20 minutes
Cooking Time: 5 minutes
Servings: 5
Ingredients:
Coconut milk, full-fat - 3 cups
Eggs - 2
Fresh orange juice - ¼ cup
Medium orange, zested - 1
Keto collagen, grass-fed - 3 scoops
Vanilla extract, unsweetened - 2 teaspoons
Erythritol sweetener - 1/8 teaspoon
Salt - 1/16 teaspoon
Gelatin, pastured - 1 ½ scoop
Water - 1 cup
Directions:
Place all the ingredients in a food processor except for the gelatin and water, pulse until smooth, then add gelatin and blend until smooth.
Divide the custard evenly between five half-pint jars and cover with their lid.
Switch on the instant pot, pour in water, insert trivet stand, place jars on it and shut the instant pot with its lid in the sealed position.
Press the 'manual' button, press '+/-' to the set the cooking time to 5 minutes and cook at high-pressure setting; when the pressure builds in the pot, the cooking timer will start.
When the instant pot buzzes, press the 'keep warm' button, do a quick pressure release and open the lid.
Carefully remove the jars, let them cool at room temperature for 15 minutes or more until they can be comfortably picked up.
Then transfer the custard jars into the refrigerator for a minimum of 4 hours and cool completely.
When ready to serve, shake the jars a few times to mix all the ingredients and then serve.
Nutrition:
Calories: 250;
Fat: 24 g;
Protein: 5 g;
Net Carbs: 2 g;
Fiber: 3 g;

Strawberry Rhubarb Custard

Preparation Time: 4 hours and 5 minutes
Cooking Time: 5 minutes
Servings: 5

Ingredients:
Coconut milk, full-fat – 27 ounces
Eggs – 2
Strawberries, fresh – ¾ cup
Rhubarb, chopped – ½ cup
Collagen, grass-fed – ¼ cup
Vanilla extract, unsweetened – 1 teaspoon
Stevia, liquid – 1/16 teaspoon
Salt – 1/16 teaspoon
Gelatin, grass-fed – 1 ½ tablespoons
Water – 1 cup
Directions:
Place all the ingredients in a food processor except for the gelatin and water, pulse until smooth, then add gelatin and blend until smooth.
Divide the custard evenly between five half-pint jars and cover with their lid.
Switch on the instant pot, pour in water, insert trivet stand, place jars on it and shut the instant pot with its lid the in the sealed position.
Press the 'manual' button, press '+/-' to set the cooking time to 5 minutes and cook at high-pressure setting; when the pressure builds in the pot, the cooking timer will start.
When the instant pot buzzes, press the 'keep warm' button, do a quick pressure release and open the lid.
Carefully remove the jars, let them cool at room temperature for 15 minutes or more until they can be comfortably picked up.
Then transfer the custard jars into the refrigerator for a minimum of 4 hours and cool completely.
When ready to serve, shake the jars a few times to mix all the ingredients and then serve.
Nutrition:
Calories: 262;
Fat: 24 g;
Protein: 5 g;
Net Carbs: 3 g;
Fiber: 3 g;

Chocolate Avocado Ice Cream

Preparation Time: 12 hours and 10 minutes
Cooking Time: 0
Servings: 6
Ingredients:
Large organic avocados, pitted – 2
Erythritol, powdered – ½ cup
Cocoa powder, organic and unsweetened – ½ cup
Drops of liquid stevia – 25
Vanilla extract, unsweetened – 2 teaspoons

Coconut milk, full-fat and unsweetened – 1 cup
Heavy whipping cream, full-fat – ½ cup
Squares of chocolate, unsweetened and chopped – 6
Directions:
Scoop out the flesh from each avocado, place it in a bowl and add vanilla, milk, and cream and blend using an immersion blender until smooth and creamy.
Add remaining ingredients except for chocolate and mix until well combined and smooth.
Fold in chopped chocolate and let the mixture chill in the refrigerator for 8 to 12 hours or until cooled.
When ready to serve, let ice cream stand for 30 minutes at room temperature, then process it using an ice cream machine as per manufacturer instruction.
Serve immediately.
Nutrition:
Calories: 216.7;
Fat: 19.4 g;
Protein: 3.8 g;
Net Carbs: 3.7 g;
Fiber: 7.4 g;

Key Lime Curd

Preparation Time: 4 hours and 30 minutes
Cooking Time: 10 minutes
Servings: 3
Ingredients:
Butter, unsalted – 3 ounces
Erythritol sweetener – 1 cup
Eggs – 2
Egg yolks – 2
Key lime juice – 2/3 cup
Key lime zest – 2 teaspoons
Water – 1 1/2 cups
Directions:
Place butter in a food processor, add sugar, blend for 2 minutes, then add eggs and yolks and continue blending for 1 minute.
Add lime juice, blend until combined and a smooth curd comes together and then pour the mixture evenly into three half-pint mason jars.
Switch on the instant pot, pour in water, insert a trivet stand, place mason jars on it and shut the instant pot with its lid the in the sealed position.
Press the 'manual' button, press '+/-' to set the cooking time to 10 minutes and cook at high-pressure setting; when the pressure builds in the pot, the cooking timer will start.
When the instant pot buzzes, press the 'keep warm' button, release pressure naturally for 10 minutes, then do a quick pressure release and open the lid.

Remove jars from the instant pot, open them, add lime zest, stir until combined and then close the jars with their lids again.
Let the jars cool at room temperature for 20 minutes, then place them in the refrigerator for 4 hours or more until chilled and curd gets thickened.
Serve straight away.
Nutrition:
Calories: 78;
Fat: 4.5 g;
Protein: 7 g;
Net Carbs: 1 g;
Fiber: 1 g;

Coconut Almond Cake

Preparation Time: 10 minutes
Cooking Time: 50 minutes
Servings: 8
Ingredients:
Almond flour – 1 cup
Shredded coconut, unsweetened – 1/2 cup
Erythritol sweetener – 1/3 cup
Baking powder – 1 teaspoon
Apple pie spice – 1 teaspoon
Eggs, whisked – 2
Butter, unsalted, melted – 1/4 cup
Heavy whipping cream – 1/2 cup and more for topping
Water – 1 cup
Directions:
Place all the ingredients in a bowl, reserving water, and stir well using a hand mixer until incorporated and a smooth batter comes together.
Take a 6-inch baking pan, spoon the prepared batter on it, then smooth the top, sprinkle with pecans and cover the pan with aluminum foil.
Switch on the instant pot, pour in water, insert a trivet stand and place pan on it.
Shut the instant pot with its lid in the sealed position, then press the 'cake' button, press '+/-' to set the cooking time to 40 minutes and cook at high-pressure setting; when the pressure builds in the pot, the cooking timer will start.
When the instant pot buzzes, press the 'keep warm' button, release pressure naturally for 10 minutes, then do a quick pressure release and open the lid. Take out the pan, uncover it, invert the pan on a plate to take out the cake and let cool for 15 minutes.
Spread cream on top of the cake, then cut into slices and serve.
Nutrition:
Calories: 236;
Fat: 23 g;
Protein: 5 g;

Net Carbs: 3 g;
Fiber: 2 g;

Spicy Almond Fat Bombs

Preparation Time: 10 minutes
Cooking Time: 4 minutes
Servings: 3
Ingredients:
¾ cup coconut oil
¼ cup almond butter
¼ cup cocoa powder
3 drops liquid stevia
⅛ teaspoon chili powder
Special equipment:
A 12-cup muffin pan
Directions:
Line a muffin pan with 12 paper liners. Keep aside.
Heat the oil in a small saucepan over low heat, then add the almond butter, cocoa powder, stevia, and chili powder. Stir to combine well.
Divide the mixture evenly among the muffin cups and keep the muffin pan in the refrigerator for 15 minutes, or until the bombs are set and firm.
Serve immediately or refrigerate to chill until ready to serve.
Nutrition:
Calories: 160
Fat: 16.8g
Total carbs: 2.0g
Fiber: 1.2g
Protein: 1.5g

Chocolate Granola Bars

Preparation Time: 10 minutes
Cooking Time: 20 minutes
Servings: 20
Ingredients:
3 ounces (85 g) almonds
3 ounces (85 g) walnuts
2 ounces (57 g) sesame seeds
2 ounces (57 g) pumpkin seeds
1 ounce (28 g) flaxseed
2 ounces (57 g) unsweetened coconut, shredded
2 ounces (57 g) dark chocolate with a minimum of 70% cocoa solids
6 tablespoons coconut oil
4 tablespoons tahini
1 teaspoon vanilla extract

2 teaspoons ground cinnamon
1 pinch sea salt
2 eggs
Directions:
Preheat your oven to 350°F (180°C).
Except for dark chocolate, process all the ingredients for granola in a food processor until they make a coarse and crumbly mixture.
Spread the granola mixture into a greased baking dish lined with parchment paper.
Bake the granola for 15 to 20 minutes in the oven until the cake turns golden brown.
Once baked, allow it to cool for 5 minutes, then remove from the baking dish.
Cut the granola cake into 24 bars using a sharp knife on a clean work surface. Set aside.
Melt the chocolate by heating in a double boiler or in the microwave. Let it cool for 5 minutes.
Serve the granola bars with the melted chocolate for dipping.
Nutrition:
Calories: 142
Fat: 17.2g
Total carbs: 7.0g
Fiber: 3.2g
Protein: 4.7g

Keto Pumpkin Spice Fat Bombs

Preparation Time: 10 minutes
Cooking Time: 0
Servings: 16
Ingredients:
½ cup butter, at room temperature
½ cup cream cheese, at room temperature
⅓ cup pumpkin purée
4 drops liquid stevia
¼ teaspoon ground nutmeg
½ teaspoon ground cinnamon
3 tablespoons chopped almonds
Directions:
Take a baking pan and line it with parchment paper. Set aside.
Place the butter and cream cheese in a small mixing bowl, and whisk well until it becomes smooth.
Pour in the pumpkin purée and blend until combined.
Add the stevia, nutmeg, cinnamon, and almonds. Stir to incorporate.
Transfer the pumpkin mixture into the pan and smooth the top with a spatula or the back of a spoon.
Keep the pan in the freezer for about 60 minutes.

Remove from the freezer and slice into 16 pieces to serve. You can preserve the fat bombs in an airtight container in the freezer until ready to eat.

Nutrition:

Calories: 80

Fat: 8.4g

Total carbs: 0.7g

Fiber: 0.1g

Protein: 0.6g

Keto Chocolate-Coconut Bites

Preparation Time: 10 minutes

Cooking Time: 3 minutes

Servings: 16

Ingredients:

⅓ cup coconut oil

¼ cup unsweetened cocoa powder

4 drops liquid stevia

Pinch sea salt

¼ cup shredded unsweetened coconut

Directions:

Line a baking dish with parchment paper. Keep it aside.

Add the coconut oil, cocoa powder, stevia, and salt in a small saucepan over low heat. Stir the mixture continuously for 2 to 3 minutes.

Once combined, stir in the shredded coconut, then transfer the mixture into the prepared baking dish.

Keep the baking dish in the refrigerator for about 30 minutes, or until the mixture is firm and set.

Slice into 16 pieces and serve immediately.

Nutrition:

Calories: 49

Fat: 5.1g

Total carbs: 1.0g

Fiber: 0.6g

Protein: 0.3g

Blueberry Lemon Cake

Preparation Time: 10 minutes

Cooking Time: 40 minutes

Servings: 4

Ingredients:

For the Cake:

2/3 cup almond flour

5 eggs

⅓ cup almond milk, unsweetened

¼ cup erythritol
2 tsp. vanilla extract
Juice of 2 lemons
1 tsp. lemon zest
½ tsp. baking soda
Pinch of salt
½ cup fresh blueberries
2 tbsp. butter, melted
For the Frosting:
½ cup heavy cream
Juice of 1 lemon
1/8 cup erythritol
Directions:
Preheat the oven to 35° F.
In a bowl, add the almond flour, eggs, and almond milk and mix well until smooth.
Add the erythritol, a pinch of salt, baking soda, lemon zest, lemon juice, and vanilla extract.
Mix and combine well.
Fold in the blueberries.
Use the butter to grease the springform pans.
Pour the batter into the greased pans.
Put on a baking sheet for even baking.
Put in the oven to bake until cooked through in the middle and slightly brown on the top, about 35 to 40 minutes.
Let cool before removing from the pan.
Mix the erythritol, lemon juice, and heavy cream. Mix well.
Serve.
Nutrition:
Calories - 274
Fat - 23.9 g
Carbs - 8.1 g
Protein - 9 g

Home Made Coconut Ice Cream

Preparation Time: 5 minutes
Cooking Time: 95 minutes
Servings: 4
Ingredients:
2 cups evaporated low-fat milk
⅓ cup low-fat condensed milk
1 cup low-fat coconut milk
½ cup stevia/xylitol/yacon syrup
2 scoops whey protein concentrate
2 tsp. sugar-free coconut extract

1 tsp. dried coconut

Directions:

Put all together the ingredients in a mixing bowl and combine well.

Heat the mixture over medium heat until it starts to bubble.

Remove from heat and allow the mixture to cool down.

Chill mixture for about an hour, then freeze in ice cream maker as outlined by the manufacturer's directions.

Nutrition:

Calories 182

Fat 1.3 g

Carbs 18 g

Protein 22.5 g

Berries with Coconut Cream

Preparation Time: 5 minutes

Cooking Time: 15 minutes

Servings: 2

Ingredients:

1 cup fat-free cream cheese

¼ cup coconut chunks

½ tsp. sugar-free coconut extract

½ cup mixed berries

3 tsp. stevia/xylitol/yacon syrup

Directions:

Beat cream cheese until fluffy.

Put the coconut chunks and stevia inside a blender and puree.

Combine using the cream cheese and set in serving plates.

Top with berries.

Serve.

Nutrition:

Calories 200

Fat 4.5 g

Carbs 17 g

Protein 23 g

Coconut Panna Cotta

Preparation Time: 5 minutes

Cooking Time: 20 minutes

Servings: 2

Ingredients:

2 cups skimmed milk

1/2 cup water

1 tsp. sugar-free coconut extract

1 envelope powdered grass-fed – organic gelatin – sugar-free

2 scoops whey protein isolate
4 tbsp. stevia/xylitol/yacon syrup
⅓ cup fresh raspberries
2 tbsp. fresh mint
Directions:
In a non-stick pan, milk, stevia, water, and coconut extract.
Bring to a boil.
Slowly add the gelatin and stir well until the mixture starts to thicken.
When ready, divide the mix among small silicon cups.
Refrigerate overnight to relax and hang up.
Remove through the fridge and thoroughly turn each cup over ahead of a serving plate.
Garnish with raspberries and fresh mint, serve and revel in!
Nutrition:
Calories 130
Fat 2.5 g
Carbs 14.4 g
Protein 29 g

Lemon & Lime Sorbet

Preparation Time: 5 minutes
Cooking Time: 140 minutes
Servings: 2
Ingredients:
1 cup water
¾ cup stevia/xylitol/yacon syrup
1 cup fresh lemon juice
2 scoops whey protein concentrate 1/2 cup lime juice
4 whole lemons or oranges cut in half, flesh removed
Directions:
Put the lake, stevia, lemon, and lime juice into a blender and puree.
Transfer to a container and freeze for about a couple of hours.
Remove from the freezer and puree once more using a blender.
Transfer to an airtight container and return to freezer.
Serve in lemon/orange cups and garnish with fresh mint.
Nutrition:
Calories 150
Fat 0.3 g
Carbs 8.5 g
Protein 25 g

Keto Vanilla Cherry Panna Cotta

Preparation Time: 10 minutes
Cooking Time: 10 minutes
Servings: 2

Ingredients:
For the vanilla layer:
1 cup heavy whipping cream
1/2 tsp vanilla extract
1 tbsp. Walnuts; roughly chopped.
2 tbsp. whole milk
1 tsp agar powder
For the cherry layer:
1 tbsp. Almonds, roughly chopped.
2 tsp cherry extract
1 cup heavy whipping cream
1 tsp agar powder
Directions:
Set the instant pot then combine all vanilla layer ingredients in the stainless steel insert. Press the *Saute* button and stir constantly. Bring it to a light simmer and then press *Cancel'* button. Transfer to a large bowl and set aside
Clean the pot and pat-dry with a kitchen paper.
Put all cherry layer ingredients and stir well. Again, bring it to a light simmer, stirring constantly
Pour about the 1/2-inch thick vanilla layer in a medium-sized glass. Put the second layer of the cherry mixture. Repeat the process until you have used both mixtures
Garnish with fresh mint and refrigerate for at least 1 hour before serving. (optional)
Nutrition:
Calories: 491 kcal
Protein: 6.82 g
Fat: 50.06 g
Carbohydrates: 5.21 g

Coconut Flan

Preparation Time: 20 minutes
Cooking Time: 9 minutes
Servings: 2
Ingredients:
2 tablespoons water
1 cup unsweetened coconut milk
3 large eggs
Pinch salt
1 cup heavy cream
¾ cup powdered erythritol, divided
2 teaspoons vanilla extract
Directions:

Whisk together ½ cup of the powdered erythritol and water in a saucepan over medium heat until it starts to darken. Divide the mixture among six small ramekins and set aside to cool.
Combine the coconut milk and cream in a saucepan and cook over medium heat until it starts to steam, whisk in the rest of the erythritol, and the vanilla extract. Beat the eggs in a mixing bowl then pour a few tablespoons of the warmed milk into it while whisking.
Put the egg mixture into the milk mixture and whisk smooth, then pour into the ramekins.
Cover the ramekins with foil and place them in the steamer insert in your Instant Pot. Pour in ½ cup water, then close and lock the lid.
Press the Manual button and adjust the timer for 9 minutes.
If the timer goes off, let the pressure vent naturally, then press Cancel.
When the pot has depressurized, open the lid.
Remove the ramekins and let the flan cool to room temperature then chill until ready to serve.
Nutrition:
Calories: 488 kcal
Protein: 18.16 g
Fat: 40.22 g
Carbohydrates: 27.75 g

Mini Vanilla Custards

Preparation Time: 20 minutes
Cooking Time: 9 minutes
Servings: 2
Ingredients:
2 tablespoons water
1 cup unsweetened almond milk
3 large eggs
Pinch salt
1 cup heavy cream
¾ cup powdered erythritol, divided
1 tablespoon vanilla extract
Directions:
Whisk together ½ cup of the powdered erythritol and water in a saucepan over medium heat until the erythritol melts.
Divide the mixture among four small ramekins and set aside to cool.
Combine the almond milk and cream in a saucepan and cook over medium heat until it starts to steam, then whisk in the rest of the erythritol and the vanilla extract.
Beat the eggs in a mixing bowl.
Whisk a few tablespoons of the milk mixture into the eggs, then whisk in the rest in a steady stream.
Cover the ramekins with foil and place them in the steamer insert in your Instant Pot.
Pour in ½ cup water, then close and lock the lid.

Press the Manual button and adjust the timer for 9 minutes.
If the timer goes off, let the pressure vent naturally, then press Cancel.
When the pot has depressurized, open the lid.
Remove the ramekins and let the custards cool for 10 minutes then serve warm.
Nutrition:
Calories: 494 kcal
Protein: 18.16 g
Fat: 40.22 g
Carbohydrates: 28.05 g

Snickerdoodles

Preparation Time: 10 minutes
Cooking Time: 10 minutes
Servings: 18
Ingredients:
1 ½ cups almond flour
6 tablespoons butter
½ cup + 2 tablespoons Sukrin Gold
1 egg
1 teaspoon pure vanilla extract
¼ teaspoon salt
¼ teaspoon ground cinnamon
¼ teaspoon ground nutmeg
⅛ teaspoon ground cloves
Directions:
Preheat your oven to 350-degrees.
Line cookie sheets with parchment paper.
In a bowl, mix the almond flour, Sukrin, and salt together.
Add in butter, vanilla, and egg.
Roll dough into 18 balls.
In another bowl, mix 2 tablespoons Sukrin with spices.
Roll cookies in it to coat.
Arrange on the cookie sheets.
Bake for 8 minutes, then check. If the sides are starting to brown and the middle looks cooked, they are done. If not, bake another 2 minutes.
Cool before serving!
Nutrition:
Calories: 94
Protein: 2 g
Carbs: 2 g
Fat: 9 g
Fiber: 0 g

Maple Almond Cake in a Jar

Preparation Time: 15 minutes
Cooking Time: 10 minutes
Servings: 4
Ingredients:
3 large eggs
¼ teaspoon salt
1 cup almond flour
1 ½ teaspoons vanilla extract
3 tablespoons sugar-free maple syrup
Directions:
Bring the trivet in the Instant Pot and add 1 cup of water.
Whisk together the almond flour, egg, sugar-free maple syrup, vanilla, and salt in a mixing bowl.
Divide the mixture among three 8-ounce jars.
Cover the jars with foil, then place on the trivet, close and lock the lid.
Press the Manual button then set the timer to 10 minutes.
If the timer goes off, do a Quick Release by pressing Cancel and switching the steam valve to "venting."
When the pot has depressurized, open the lid.
Remove the jars and let them cool a little before serving.
Nutrition:
Calories: 73 kcal
Protein: 4.06 g
Fat: 5.32 g
Carbohydrates: 2.59 g

Keto Almond Butter Fudge Slices

Preparation Time: 10 minutes
Cooking Time: 0
Servings: 36
Ingredients:
1 cup coconut oil, at room temperature
10 drops liquid stevia
1 cup almond butter
1 pinch sea salt
¼ cup heavy whipping cream
Directions:
Take a baking dish and line it with parchment paper. Set aside.
Whisk together the coconut oil, stevia, almond butter, salt, and heavy cream in a medium bowl until the mixture becomes smooth.
Transfer the mixture into the prepared baking dish. Smooth the top with the back of a spoon or spatula.
Keep the dish in the refrigerator for 2 hours or until the fudge is totally set and firm.

Remove from the refrigerator and slice into 36 pieces to serve.
Nutrition:
Calories: 100
Fat: 10.2g
Total carbs: 1.3g
Fiber: 0.7g
Protein: 1.5g

Almond Flour Shortbread Cookies

Preparation Time: 10 minutes
Cooking Time: 10 minutes
Servings: 18
Ingredients:
½ cup butter, at room temperature, plus more for greasing the baking sheet
1 teaspoon vanilla extract
½ cup Swerve
1½ cups almond flour
½ cup ground hazelnuts
1 pinch sea salt
Directions:
Start by mixing the butter, vanilla extract, and Swerve in a medium mixing bowl until well combined.
Add the almond four, salt, and ground hazelnuts. Stir until you get a firm dough.
Shape the mixture into a 2-inch cylinder. Cover it with plastic wrap and let rest in the refrigerator for about 30 minutes until it's firm.
Preheat the oven to 350°F (180ºC) and grease a parchment paper-lined baking sheet with butter. Keep it aside.
Remove the almond flour dough from the refrigerator. On a clean work surface, slice it into 18 pieces and put them on the prepared baking sheet.
Bake for 8 to 10 minutes or until firm and lightly browned in color.
Transfer to a wire rack to cool completely before serving.
Nutrition:
Calories: 116
Fat: 10.7g
Total carbs: 2.6g
Fiber: 0.4g
Protein: 2.8g

Healthy Vanilla-Almond Ice Pops

Preparation Time: 10 minutes
Cooking Time: 5 minutes
Servings: 8
Ingredients:
2 cups unsweetened almond milk

1 vanilla bean, halved lengthwise
1 cup heavy whipping cream
1 cup unsweetened coconut, shredded
Directions:
Heat the almond milk in a saucepan over medium heat, then add the vanilla bean, and heavy cream. Mix well and bring the mixture to a simmer.
Reduce the heat to low and simmer for 5 minutes more.
Turn off the heat and allow the mixture to cool.
Remove the vanilla bean from the mixture, then scrape out the seeds out of the pod with a knife, throwing the seeds into the mixture.
Add the shredded coconut and pour the liquid between the ice pop molds evenly.
Place the ice molds in the refrigerator for 4 hours until ready to serve.
Nutrition:
Calories: 125
Fat: 10.9g
Total carbs: 5.0g
Fiber: 0.9g
Protein: 2.6g

Low-Carb Raspberry Cheesecake

Preparation Time: 10 minutes
Cooking Time: 30 minutes
Servings: 12
Ingredients:
⅔ cup coconut oil, melted
½ cup cream cheese, at room temperature
6 eggs, whisked
3 tablespoons granulated sweetener
½ teaspoon baking powder
1 teaspoon vanilla extract
¾ cup raspberries
Directions:
Preheat the oven to 350°F (180ºC) and line a baking dish with parchment paper. Keep it aside.
Place the coconut oil and cream cheese in a large mixing bowl and whisk the mixture with an electric mixer until smooth.
Add the whisked eggs to the bowl, stopping once to scrape down the sides of the bowl with a spatula.
Fold in the sweetener, baking powder, and vanilla extract, and blend well.
Transfer the mixture into the lined baking dish and smooth the top with a spatula. Top with the raspberries.
Bake for 28 to 30 minutes or until the center is set and firm.
Once the cheesecake has cooled completely, slice them into 12 squares to serve.

Nutrition:
Calories: 210
Fat: 20.4g
Total carbs: 1.9g
Fiber: 0.5g
Protein: 5.2g

Keto Lava Cake

Preparation Time: 15 minutes
Cooking Time: 10 minutes
Servings: 6
Ingredients:
1 tablespoon melted butter, for greasing the ramekins
2 ounces (57 g) dark chocolate with a minimum of 70% cocoa solids
2 ounces (57 g) butter
¼ teaspoon vanilla extract
3 eggs
Special equipment:
4 to 6 small ramekins
Directions:
Preheat your oven to 400°F (205°C) and lightly grease 4 to 6 small ramekins with 1 tablespoon melted butter.
Cut the chocolate into small pieces on your cutting board. Add the chocolate and butter to a double broiler, and heat until they are melted. Mix well.
Add the vanilla to the chocolate mixture, then allow the mixture to cool.
Beat all the eggs in a mixing bowl for 3 minutes until fluffy, then add the chocolate mixture. Stir to combine.
Divide the mixture among the greased ramekins. Bake all the ramekins in the preheated oven for 5 minutes.
Remove from the oven and cool for 5 minutes before enjoying.
Nutrition:
Calories: 197
Fat: 17.8g
Total carbs: 4.9g
Fiber: 1.0g
Protein: 5.4g

Coco Avocado Truffles

Preparation Time: 35 minutes
Cooking Time: 0
Servings: 20
Ingredients:
1 ripe avocado, chopped
½ teaspoon vanilla extract

½ lime zest
1 pinch salt
5 ounces (142 g) dark chocolate with a minimum of 80% cocoa solids, finely chopped
1 tablespoon coconut oil
1 tablespoon unsweetened cocoa powder
Directions:
In a bowl, thoroughly mix the avocado flesh with vanilla extract with an electric hand mixer until it forms a smooth mixture.
Add the lime zest and a pinch of salt, then mix well. Set aside.
Mix and melt the chocolate with coconut oil in a double broiler or by heating in the microwave.
Add the chocolate mixture to the avocado mash. Blend well until a smooth batter forms.
Refrigerate this batter for 30 minutes until firm.
Scoop portions of the batter (about 2 teaspoons in size) and shape into small truffle balls with your hands, then roll each truffle ball in the cocoa powder. Serve immediately.
Nutrition:
Calories: 61
Fat: 5.2g
Total carbs: 4.3g
Fiber: 1.6g
Protein: 0.8g

Chocolate Chip Cookies

Preparation Time: 5 minutes
Cooking Time: 24 minutes
Servings: 6
Ingredients:
Almond flour – ½ cup and 2 tablespoons
Shredded coconut, unsweetened – 6 tablespoons
Salt – 1/4 teaspoon
Swerve sweetener – 1/4 cup
Baking powder – 1/2 teaspoon
Chocolate chips, unsweetened – 2 1/2 tablespoons
Yacon syrup – 1 teaspoon
Vanilla extract, unsweetened – 1/4 teaspoon
Butter, unsalted and softened – 1/4 cup
Egg, organic – 1
Directions:
Switch on the oven, set it to 375 degrees F and preheat.
Place flour in a bowl, add shredded coconut along with salt and baking powder and stir until mixed.
Place butter in another bowl, add sweetener and yacon syrup and beat until combined.

Then beat egg and vanilla until blended and then beat in flour mixture, ½ cup at a time, until incorporated and the smooth dough comes together.
Fold chocolate chips into the dough and then shape into 1 ½ inch balls.
Take a large baking sheet, line with parchment paper, then arrange balls on it, 2-inch apart and press them slightly with the heel of your hand to ¼-inch thick cookie.
Place the baking sheet into the oven and bake cookies for 15 minutes or until nicely golden brown and slightly firm.
When done, remove the baking sheet from the oven and let the cookies cool completely, then serve.
Nutrition:
Calories: 238;
Fat: 21.6 g;
Protein: 4.4 g;
Net Carbs: 4.8 g;
Fiber: 3.4 g;

Blueberry Muffins

Preparation Time: 25 minutes
Cooking Time: 20 minutes
Servings: 6
Ingredients:
Coconut flour - ⅓ cup
Golden flaxseed meal - 1 ½ tablespoon
Erythritol sweetener - 4 ½ tablespoons
Baking powder - 1 teaspoon
Baking soda - ¼ teaspoon
Sea salt - ⅛ teaspoon
Almond milk, unsweetened - 1/3 cup
Eggs, beaten - 2
Butter, unsalted, melted - 1 ½ tablespoon
Vanilla extract, unsweetened - 1 teaspoon
Blueberries, fresh - 1/3 cup
Water - 1 cup
Heavy cream - as needed for topping
Directions:
Place flour in a large bowl, add flaxseed, baking powder, baking soda, sweetener and salt, and mix until well combined.
Crack eggs in another bowl, add vanilla, butter and milk and whisk until smooth.
Gradually mix the milk mixture into flour mixture until incorporated and smooth and then fold in berries until just mixed.
Switch on the instant pot, pour in water, insert a trivet stand and line with a 10-inch sheet of aluminum foil.

Spoon six silicone cupcake liners with muffin batter until ¾ full, then place the cupcakes on the lined trivet stand and cover the muffins with another sheet of aluminum foil.
Shut the instant pot with its lid in the sealed position, then press the 'manual' button, press '+/-' to set the cooking time to 20 minutes and cook at high-pressure setting; when the pressure builds in the pot, the cooking timer will start.
When the instant pot buzzes, press the 'keep warm' button, release pressure naturally for 10 minutes, then do a quick pressure release and open the lid.
Remove and discard the foil, lift out muffins and let cool on a wire rack for 15 minutes.
Pipe cream on top and serve straight away.
Nutrition:
Calories: 130;
Fat: 11 g;
Protein: 3 g;
Net Carbs: 1.5 g;
Fiber: 2 g;

Peanut Butter Mousse

Preparation Time: 5 minutes
Cooking Time: 0
Servings: 4
Ingredients:
½ cup heavy whipping cream
4 oz cream cheese, softened
¼ cup natural peanut butter
¼ cup powdered Swerve sweetener
½ tsp vanilla extract
Directions:
Beat ½ cup cream in a medium bowl with a hand mixer until it forms peaks.
Beat cream cheese with peanut butter in another bowl until creamy.
Stir in vanilla, a pinch of salt, and sweetener to the peanut butter mix and combine until smooth.
Fold in the prepared whipped cream and mix well until fully incorporated.
Divide the mousse into 4 serving glasses.
Garnish as desired.
Enjoy.
Nutrition:
Calories 290
Total Fat 21.5 g
Saturated Fat 15.2 g
Cholesterol 12.1 mg
Sodium 9 mg
Total Carbs 6.5 g
Sugar 1.2 g

Fiber 0.4 g
Protein 6.2 g

Cookie Ice Cream

Preparation Time: 5 minutes
Cooking Time: 2 hours
Servings: 2
Ingredients:
Cookie Crumbs
¾ cup almond flour
¼ cup cocoa powder
¼ tsp baking soda
¼ cup erythritol
½ tsp vanilla extract
1 ½ tbsp coconut oil, softened
1 large egg, room temperature
Pinch of salt
Ice Cream
2 ½ cups whipping cream
1 tbsp vanilla extract
½ cup erythritol
½ cup almond milk, unsweetened
Directions:
Preheat your oven at 300 degrees F and layer a 9-inch baking pan with wax paper.
Whisk almond flour with baking soda, cocoa powder, salt, and erythritol in a medium bowl.
Stir in coconut oil and vanilla extract then mix well until crumbly.
Whisk in egg and mix well to form the dough.
Spread this dough in the prepared pan and bake for 20 minutes in the preheated oven.
Allow the crust to cool then crush it finely into crumbles.
Beat cream in a large bowl with a hand mixer until it forms a stiff peak.
Stir in erythritol and vanilla extract then mix well until fully incorporated.
Pour in milk and blend well until smooth.
Add this mixture to an ice cream machine and churn as per the machine's instructions.
Add cookie crumbles to the ice cream in the machine and churn again.
Place the ice cream in a sealable container and freeze for 2 hours.
Scoop out the ice cream and serve.
Enjoy.
Nutrition:
Calories 214
Total Fat 19 g
Saturated Fat 5.8 g
Cholesterol 15 mg
Sodium 123 mg

Total Carbs 6.5 g
Sugar 1.9 g
Fiber 2.1 g
Protein 6.5 g

Pumpkin Pecan Ice Cream

Preparation Time: 4 hours and 5 minutes
Cooking Time: 0
Servings: 4
Ingredients:
½ cup cottage cheese
½ cup pumpkin puree
1 tsp pumpkin spice
2 cups unsweetened coconut milk
½ tsp xanthan gum
3 large egg yolks
1/3 cup erythritol
20 drops liquid stevia
1 tsp maple extract
½ cup chopped pecans, toasted
2 tbsp salted butter
Directions:
Add butter to a saucepan and place it over low heat until butter turns brown.
Whisk the remaining ingredients in a separate bowl using a hand mixer.
Churn this mixture in the ice cream mixture as per the machine's instructions.
Toss pecans with butter then add them to the ice cream.
Churn again then freeze for 4 hours.
Enjoy.
Nutrition:
Calories 331
Total Fat 38.5 g
Saturated Fat 19.2 g
Cholesterol 141 mg
Sodium 283 mg
Total Carbs 9.2 g
Sugar 3 g
Fiber 1 g
Protein 2.1 g

Mocha Ice Cream

Preparation Time: 2 hours and 5 minutes
Cooking Time: 0
Servings: 2
Ingredients:

1 cup coconut milk
¼ cup heavy whipping cream
2 tbsp erythritol
15 drops liquid stevia
2 tbsp unsweetened cocoa powder
1 tbsp instant coffee
¼ tsp xanthan gum
Directions:
Whisk everything except xanthan gum in a bowl using a hand mixer.
Slowly add xanthan gum and stir well to make a thick mixture.
Churn the mixture in an ice cream machine as per the machine's instructions.
Freeze it for 2 hours then garnish with mint and instant coffee.
Serve.
Nutrition:
Calories 267
Total Fat 44.5 g
Saturated Fat 17.4 g
Cholesterol 153 mg
Sodium 217 mg
Total Carbs 8.4 g
Sugar 2.3 g
Fiber 1.3 g
Protein 3.1 g

Conclusion

Keto can be a great option for people looking to shed extra weight that is stored in their bodies as fat. Ketosis is the process of the body using fats instead of glucose for energy. The liver can take fats and break them down into ketones, which can be used by both the body and the brain as a fuel source. To get the body away from using sugars, however, a person has to severely limit the amount and type of carbs they consume so the body can burn through its glucose stores and start working on the fat stores. This is why it can be so important to stay diligent on the diet once started; otherwise, a person might not see their desired results.

For people who are ready to dedicate themselves 100% to the keto diet, there are various forms of it that can match any person's lifestyle and goals. The standard keto option is best for people trying the diet for the first time because it can be the quickest way to get into ketosis and reap the immediate benefits. There are also cyclical and targeted keto for people who might not be willing to follow the strict diet every day. These options give people an opportunity to consume carbs on certain days based on their own personal plans.

There are many benefits to starting the keto diet beyond just losing weight. Keto can also help people improve their heart health by reducing bad fats and forcing the body to work through fats it has stored, possibly in dangerous places like arteries. It can also help people with certain types of epilepsy reduce seizures by switching the brain onto ketone power. Keto can also help women with PCOS regain their health by promoting weight loss and helping to balance their hormones, which can be a cause of the condition. It can even help clear up acne in some people by reducing blood sugar, which can improve skin conditions.

It is not difficult to switch to and stick to a Keto diet. What is actually difficult is adhering to strict rules and guidelines. As long as you maintain the Fats : Protein : Carbs ratio, you'll lose weight fast. It's a no-brainer. And quite unbecoming that many have deviated from this core principle of the Keto diet. The simple formula is to increase the fat and protein content in your meals and snacks while reducing your carb intake. You must restrict your carb intake to reach and remain in Ketosis. Different people achieve Ketosis with varying amounts of carb intake. Generally, it is easy to reach and stay in Ketosis when you decrease your carb intake to not more than 20grams.

Keeping keto long term can seem difficult for beginners who are just getting used to the mechanics of the diet, but it is not so difficult once they are acclimated to the keto lifestyle. Planning out meals and snacks can help people keep up keto longer because it takes some of the work and thinking out of dieting. A person can simply grab what they need and go. And if the standard keto doesn't work for someone long term, they can refer to the other keto styles to find one that will work for them beyond the initial diet.

CPSIA information can be obtained
at www.ICGtesting.com
Printed in the USA
LVHW060020210221
679536LV00009B/308

9 787830 646929